90-DAY HABIT TRANSFORMATION
The Essential Guide to Sustainable
Fitness, Nutrition, And Personal Well-Being

By Michael S. Parker

eBook
ISBN-13: 978-1-7350614-4-3

Paperback
ISBN-13: 978-1-7350614-2-9

Hardback
ISBN-13: 978-1-7350614-3-6

Audiobook
ISBN-13: 978-1-7350614-5-0

Library of Congress Control Number:
2022922989

Cover and Graphics by Turning Heads Designs
www.turningheadsdesigns.com

This book is dedicated to all my clients and those who struggle with fitness and nutrition but never give up.

Contents

PART I **15**

ABOUT THE AUTHOR **17**

HOW I SHAPED MY PHILOSOPHY **19**

HOW TO USE THIS BOOK **27**

PART I OVERVIEW 29

PART II OVERVIEW 29

PART III OVERVIEW 29

TRANSFORMATION SCHEDULE 30

Chapter One **39**

THE BEAUTY & FITNESS LIE **39**

Beauty Lies 39

The Skinny Lie 40

The Zero Blemish Lie 43

The Fashion Lie 45

Fitness Lies 46

The Gimmick Lie 47

The Nutrition Lie 48

The Duration Lie 50

A Note on The Body Positive Movement 53

Chapter Keynotes 55

Chapter Two **57**

THE BASICS OF HABIT **57**

Habits Are Efficiency Adaptations 57

Habit and Resistance - Oscillation 59

Habit and Resistance – Selective Knowledge 61

Habit and Resistance – Return Versus Effort 65

Habit and Resistance – Fear 67

Chapter Keynotes 75

Chapter Three **79**

THE 30X3+10 RULE **79**

Attitude = 30% 81

Nutrition = 30%......................................86

Activity = 30% 90

Genetics = 10% 91

Chapter Keynotes 97

Chapter Four **101**

STAGES OF CHANGE **101**

Precontemplation 102

Contemplation 102

Preparation 103

Action...103

Maintenance.......................................104

Chapter Keynotes 105

Chapter Five **107**

WELLNESS CONSCIOUSNESS **107**

Stage One: Careless Unconsciousness...............108

Stage Two: Conscious Realization..................108

Stage Three: Conscious Action 110

Stage Four: Conscious Maintenance................111

Wellness Action and Consequence..................111

Constructive Action 112

Destructive Action 112

Behavior Intensity (Y) 113

Behavior Duration (X) 113

Chapter Keynotes 116

Chapter Six **119**

THE POWER OF CONSCIOUS RESPONSE **119**

Behavior Instigation 122

Instigator Acquisition 124

Instigator Comprehension 125

Habit Comparison 126

Conscious Response 127

Positive Events May Be Instigators 129

Chapter Keynotes 129

Chapter Seven **133**

DEVELOPING INTENDED OUTCOMES **133**

The F.I.N.D Principle 135

Focus your Passion 136

Invest in your Personality...................................... 139

Navigate with Agility 140

Develop Perseverance.. 141

Chapter Keynotes 142

Chapter Eight **147**

SEVEN INTELLIGENT PERSONALITY TRAITS **147**

Intelligent Self-Awareness 147

Intelligent Trust... 148

Intelligent Integrity 150

Intelligent Courage.. 151

Intelligent Humor.. 152

Intelligent Emotional Sense 152

Intelligent Discipline 154

Chapter Keynotes 155

Chapter Nine **161**

SETTING REALISTIC EXPECTATIONS AND GOALS **161**

Setting Expectations 161

The Motivation Myth 164

Limiting Beliefs... 166

5 Steps for Setting Goals 167

Chapter Keynotes 178

Chapter Ten **181**

SETTING PERSONAL & PROFESSIONAL BOUNDARIES ... **181**

Personal Boundaries 183

Silent Boundaries 184

Formal Boundaries...................................... 185

Boundaries for Pets 187

Professional Boundaries 187

Work-life Balance 188

Chapter Keynotes 188

PART II **193**

Chapter Eleven **195**

90-DAY HABIT **195**

TRANSFORMATION WORKBOOK **195**

Week One Action 196

Week Two Action....................................... 196

Week Three Action 200

Week Four Action 204

Week Five Action 206

Week Six Action 207

Week Seven Action 209

Week Eight Action 211

Week Nine Action 211

Week Ten Action 216

Week Eleven Action 218

Week Twelve Action 219

Week Forever 220

PART III **223**

Chapter Twelve **225**

WHERE TO START WITH NUTRITION **225**

How to Read a Nutrition Label 229

Carbohydrates: The Truth 231

Protein: The Truth 242

Fat: The Truth 250

Hydration 257

Chapter Thirteen **260**

PRACTICAL NUTRITION CONCEPTS **261**

Commit to Yourself and the Plan 261

Clean House 262

Choose Nutrition Over Calories 262

Pre-Plan & Time Balanced Meals 263

Add Variety and Keep It Fresh 263

Chapter Fourteen **267**

WHERE TO START WITH FITNESS **267**

Weight Training Fundamentals 267

The 6 Levels of Fitness Hierarchy......................................267

Mobility..268

Flexibility...268

Stability...269

Strength...269

Power...269

Skill..270

Acute Variables Basics 270

Posture & Form: It's Not How Much, It's How You Lift ...272

Recovery Basics: Active and Passive Recovery Is Key 273

Common Exercise Terms and Modality Basics 274

5 Reasons Women Should Be Weight Training.................284

3 Reasons to Stop Weighing Yourself Frequently............287

Top 5 Mistakes People Make at The Gym 289

Chapter Fifteen **301**

OVERCOMING FEELINGS OF DEFEAT............................ **301**

Stop and Acknowledge 302

Set Micro Goals..302

Enjoy the Journey 303

Recount Your Success 303

Control Your Reactions 303

Chapter Sixteen **307**

OVERCOMING FITNESS FAILURE **307**

Select & Hire a Professional Personal Trainer or Coach. .307

Join A Small Group Training Program. 308

Get Involved with Group Exercise Classes. 309

Hiking, Walking, and Outdoors. 309

Get Involved with Team or Individual Sports.................310

Chapter Seventeen 313

HOW TO CHOOSE A PERSONAL TRAINER OR COACH ... 313

    Live Personal Training Advantages.. 313

    Online Coaching and Training Advantages......................... 315

Chapter Eighteen 319

HOW TO CHOOSE A FITNESS FACILITY 319

    Corporate Chain Gyms & Franchises............................... 319

    Boutique Personal Training Studios 320

    Olympic Style Gyms.. 321

    Yoga, Pilates, and Mind-Body Studios........................... 322

    Luxury Brand or Country Clubs 322

Chapter Nineteen 325

HOW TO OVERCOME HOLIDAY TEMPTATIONS............ 325

    Set A Personal Calorie Limit 325

    Choose Only Your Favorite Foods 325

    Keep Active 326

    Manage Your Alcohol Consumption 326

    Commit to a Lifelong Wellness Plan.............................. 327

Chapter Twenty 329

HOW TO STAY ON TRACK WHEN TRAVELING 329

    Commit Unconditionally to Your Plan............................ 329

    Prepare Snacks for Transit Time 329

    Research Destination Meal and Fitness Options............. 330

    Prioritize Some Form of Daily Exercise.......................... 330

    Remain Hydrated and Well Rested 331

    Balance Indulgence with Moderation 331

Chapter Twenty-One.. 335

HOW TO KEEP YOUR RESOLUTIONS 335

Why Resolutions Fail...335

Be Specific and Realistic...336

Set A Schedule 336

Work Toward Progress, Not Perfection 336

Start Practicing Positive Affirmations 337

Change Your Habits, Change Your Life.............................337

COMPREHENSIVE MEAL PLANS 352

1,200 CALORIE MEAL PLAN OUTLINES...........................353

1,600 CALORIE MEAL PLAN OUTLINES...........................361

2,000 CALORIE MEAL PLAN OUTLINES...........................369

2,400 CALORIE MEAL PLAN OUTLINES...........................377

FOOD EXCHANGE LIST 385

ACKNOWLEDGEMENTS...387

PART I
HABIT, BEHAVIOR, AND MINDSET

ABOUT THE AUTHOR

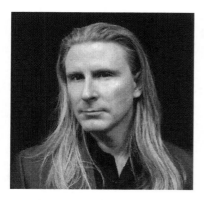 For over two decades, Michael S. Parker has worked as a fitness professional and executive-level manager. He has earned multiple credentials from the National Academy of Sports Medicine, National Exercise & Sports Trainers Association, and the Spencer Institute. He is a Certified Master Personal Trainer, Lifestyle & Weight Management Coach, and Functional Movement Specialist.

He also holds a business degree from the University of Phoenix. Michael is a former college instructor and consultant to the Advanced Personal Training and Exercise Science program offered by Bryan University. Further, he is an advisor, author, and consultant to multiple fitness companies and publications in the United States.

In 2019, 2020, 2021, and 2022, Michael was ranked as one of the top online personal trainers and habit coaches in the world by Consumers Advocate and has been featured on multiple fitness blogs, podcasts, and other media. He is an avid outdoors person and spends much of his time backpacking, mountaineering, snowboarding, motorcycling, and traveling.

Michael is the Founder and CEO of Forge Fitness and Nutrition Coaching. Forge provides highly custom online fitness and nutrition coaching services designed to accommodate all fitness levels. Forge works with individuals and corporations to improve habit-based wellness strategies in over 60 countries around the world and counting.

Here is an overview of Michaels primary credentials:

CERTIFIED PERSONAL TRAINER
National Academy of Sports Medicine

CERTIFIED FITNESS NUTRITION SPECIALIST
National Academy of Sports Medicine

CERTIFIED PERSONAL TRAINER
National Exercise and Sports Trainer Association

CERTIFIED FITNESS NUTRITION COACH
National Exercise and Sports Trainer Association

CERTIFIED LIFESTYLE & WEIGHT MANAGEMENT SPECIALIST
National Exercise and Sports Trainer Association

CERTIFIED SPORTS INJURY SPECIALIST
National Exercise and Sports Trainer Association

CERTIFIED PHYSIQUE & FIGURE TRAINING SPECIALIST
National Exercise and Sports Trainer Association

CERTIFIED FUNCTIONAL MOVEMENT SPECIALIST
Functional Movement Systems

CERTIFIED ONLINE COACH
Spencer Institute

CERTIFIED SMALL BUSINESS COACH
Spencer Institute

HOW I SHAPED MY PHILOSOPHY

As a young man, I always had a curiosity to work in the wellness industry. I sensed a fitness career would be fun and double as a method of providing for myself and my family while helping others. I found it attractive from a symbiotic standpoint, and that fostered my passion to add value to my sphere of influence.

Because a few of my friends worked for a large chain of fitness centers in the late 1990s, I gained some inside information about the environment and earning potential of fitness club managers and executives before I started in the year 2000.

The combination of what I initially perceived to be a positive environment, potential career growth, and opportunity to make a difference in the community by way of health and fitness, caused a strong magnetism to the industry.

At the time this book was published, I had been working as a fitness professional for over two decades, and like most career fitness pros, I started in the aforementioned corporate chain gyms.

This early experience gave me the tidal wave of volume one would expect from a San Francisco Bay Area gym company allowing me to interact with tens of thousands of people for years as a trainer and manager.

I was fortunate to work with other talented fitness professionals, learned from my own experiences, and by collaborating with other trainers, managers, and executives I added to my collective experience.

I believe continuing education is critical for serious fitness professionals, so I have earned multiple credentials from the National Academy of Sports Medicine, the National Exercise Sports Trainer Association and I am a Functional Movement Specialist.

Sometime in 2007, I realized that for folks to see any reasonable and long-term results with fitness and nutrition, they would need to address the root cause behaviors that detract from a healthy lifestyle, so I shifted my education toward life coaching and other behavior studies.

This book is a collected review of my professional experiences and the results of my study of habit formation and alteration. Essentially, these opinions are the culmination of over twenty years working with people in arguably the most challenging modern personal endeavor, which is to maintain balanced fitness and nutrition as a sustainable lifestyle in commonly sedentary work environments, high calorie, and low nutrition food options, and a growing desire for minimal effort with maximum return.

On my journey through these experiences, I found that fitness and nutrition success is really all about finding your particular "combination" like a lock. Once you find your personal code, then it is as simple as lining up the components and turning the key. But I instinctively knew there was more to wellness management than just diet or exercise.

Yet, I found that in many ways, the media and many companies producing products and services over-simplified what it takes to remain fit in the modern world while simultaneously convoluting reasonable fitness and nutrition outcome expectations.

This simplification and convolution are intended to sell products, fad diets, programs, or gimmicks. I wanted to get away from all the marketing hype and fitness commodity and find real solutions.

It was during these few years I associated attitude-based behavior change, or habit formation, into the fitness and nutrition concepts found in this book.

In 2007, I began working as a consultant to Bryan University's degree program for Advanced Fitness & Nutrition Sciences while building my personal training and consulting businesses.

The combination of my involvement with academia and connecting with people struggling to achieve and then maintain fitness sparked my philosophy on sustainable fitness & nutrition practices.

A good blend of science and empathy toward individual needs as it relates to long-term results became the cornerstone of my coaching style. But for all the technical exercise programming and creative nutrition, I was dismayed by the massive amount of fitness failure people experience daily.

Like I mentioned above, in our modern world of convenience and abundance, we have become conditioned to expect instant gratification and put forth minimal effort.

The inspiration for this book came from the desire to clear the clutter related to fitness and nutrition concepts and provide a roadmap for sustainable behavior change. However, while the process for this is based on 90 days, real success and continued improvement will come from a lifetime of personal attention to your activity level, food management, and adherence to positive behaviors that produce lasting results.

The next 90 days are only the foundation for a lifelong execution of principles and health habits that work for you. I have also developed several systems to bring elevated consciousness to the forefront and intercede learned negative automatic responses, formed from bad reactionary habits.

The concept of relationships and internal and external trust are an arching theme in my philosophy, and you will see examples reoccurring throughout this book.

Habit alteration requires a realistic assessment of the environment, so one will understand the characteristics that must be possessed to achieve success. We must fortify our resolve and continue the proactive movement necessary to illuminate the areas of ourselves that are undesirable and forge who we want to be. That statement is a prime motivation for taking the time and energy to write this book and share.

But first, let's address the wide fitness industry in general as I am a massive critic of it and social media influence. Like thousands of other fitness professionals, I became aware quickly that a large majority of the fitness industry can be obnoxiously immature, and true quality solutions or competent education often gets lost in the overwhelming amount of misinformation.

Worse still, an unveiled greed prevails through the industry that has devalued the role of a fitness professional through marketing tricks, gimmicks, and product infomercials.

I became frustrated with the singular focus of profits over solutions, and the consumers paid the price. To be clear, I have an entrepreneurial spirit and affirm profit is not the problem, but the way it is pursued can be.

Worse yet, the fitness industry and media machines have now conditioned the market to flit from fad to fad and invest in fraudulent pills, powders, and dangerous eating habits or surgeries.

Subsequently, most people have now developed an unhealthy relationship with food, despise exercise, and have unrealistic expectations. This has resulted in a mass absolution from addressing the root cause to make positive personal changes as individuals. Many people are just unhappy and ready to blame or look for the next shortcut.

Instead of turning their focus inward to solve the issue, people now blame the diet fad they tried and failed, genetics, the pill they wasted money on, or just screw it and have parts of their body surgically removed. What the hell is going on here?

People would rather elect to permanently destroy their digestive system by removing parts of their anatomy instead of changing a habit. Unless a physician feels it is medically relevant, we should not be cutting parts of ourselves off. It's kind of a basic life rule. I will come back to consumer behavior in a few paragraphs, so hold tight.

I am calling for a rebuke on those in the wide fitness industry who continue to commoditize and reduce the value of total wellness and erode the market's perception of that value.

This includes the club owners and industry players that use cut-rate marketing, price manipulation, low-value services in exchange for volume, slashed personal training pricing, poor customer service, questionable sales practices, unprofessional staff, uneducated trainers, and inferior managers.

Mostly, I am disgusted with the garbage pedaled on social media platforms from false trainers or so-called "models" and "influencers" adding to the confusion and get-fit-quick schemes.

Infomercials also use predatory marketing to snare the desperate and confused into the next low-effort gimmick. Words like "science" are thrown around, and even some medical doctors have sold out and aligned themselves with the money, not the mission for sustainable change.

The overwhelming focus on producing revenue is so intense and relentless it challenges willpower to remain in the industry for some, while others experience a collapse of integrity simply to meet a revenue goal or gain a false influencer status on social media.

I noticed the industry's perpetual deviation toward fad or any other potential money sources that could be twisted and yanked in a clumsy troll-like eagerness to bash, wring and squeeze every drop of revenue from the market as possible.

To develop as a rounded fitness professional, I would have to keep a solid foundation in business fundamentals, proven science, fad avoidance, and genuine communication, especially if I were to combat the flood of inaccurate information and misguided advice spewing from every corner of this expanding industry.

As it is, I struggle to dispel misinformation or even keep up with or effectively negate the greedy, absurd, or down-right silly products or notions pedaled to the desperate public and microsphere of my clients. And it is the predatory approach and self-actualizing stereotype I reprehend about the fitness industry.

While I cannot and will never be a true expert in this vast subject of all aspects of wellness, I will most certainly never stop learning and will keep an open mind.

This means that if a new product or worthwhile approach emerges, I will openly consider it, contrast, and compare and make a value judgment on its merits. As a fitness professional, there will be many programs, methods, theories, and even equipment I encounter.

Questioning the validity, safety, or sustainability of a product or service is prudent and I approach each new idea with the mind of a student. Once I assess the new product or program, I compare it to the fundamental mechanisms of fitness and nutrition.

Then, I cautiously form a loose opinion and test. I do this so I am constantly expanding my capacity, and therefore, my clients get the best service based on knowledge and experience. At the end of the day, a kettlebell is just a cannonball with a handle and not a miracle.

Now let's circle back to the issue I see with the consumer and know this; I will reiterate this issue throughout the book. In general, the public is deconditioned, sedentary, and dissatisfied with their level of wellness. Appearance and body issues aside, people are not feeling well, have less energy, are more susceptible to injury and illness, and lack general conditioning.

Now add those conditions to poor body image and repeated fitness failure and you have a typical profile of many of your very own neighbors, friends, and family.

People in your circle might even describe you this way at one point in your life or even today. The blinding pace of expanding fitness products and services is exhausting. Between the many tendrils of the health and wellness sector along with the general degradation of quality content on the internet, folks are confused.

It seems there is just too much information and emotional capital invested by individuals and corporations alike to stop and consider approach and ethics.

In addition, many ideas toted as new, are simply old products or methods dressed up and rebranded. Kettlebells are an ancient modality; suspension training techniques are centuries old and high-intensity training programs are not a modern revelation.

Just research the conditioning methods of historic gladiators and soldiers and you will see familiar exercises and training modalities. The nature of the fitness industry allows us to just slap a few pretty colors on an old box, make a promotional video with attractive people and beat-driven music while simply regurgitating tired ideas, and resell as if it were innovative and revolutionary.

Again, this works because the public is desperate for fitness solutions, and dare, I say again, they want to invest minimal effort. Therefore, fads or other products with enough glitter will sell because of the quick-fix-low-investment desire of many consumers. All this trash in the fitness and nutrition market is the product of consumer distress and laziness. I know, not a popular topic, but it is certainly true.

People want it now and they don't want to work for it, especially long term. When I finally submitted to this realization, I decided where to place my energy and how to best serve my community and clients.

For me to help solve this problem, I concluded my ability to understand sustainable habit formation and proper application of fitness and nutrition concepts would be critical to my competency and, conversely, the success of my clients by way of my expanding expertise.

I also learned that my target audience is narrow compared to most coaches and trainers selling products and services online. I appeal to a smaller market because I do not make false yet enticing promises or exaggerated claims about what it takes to succeed.

I would rather have a small and intimate group of clients to whom I add tremendous value versus being just another peddler of gimmicks with a large audience. This is also true for my social media presence, which I have little use for and spend very little time cultivating. For me personally, it's a complete waste of time and energy.

Anyhow, my career experience with the fitness industry, client behavior observations, and the nature of the modern world of incredible abundance has defined my philosophy. I believe in providing quality programs for each client based on their unique situation with an emphasis on root cause habit alteration. Fitness is more about total well-being and less about aesthetics.

Proper nutrition, strength, and endurance fortify our health and give us the power to meet life's adventures head-on. A figure to be proud of is simply a lovely byproduct of fitness and nutrition management. I understand appearance is important, but our bodies will degrade over time, we must work to be the best version of ourselves in habit, exercise, nutrition, and attitude every day.

HOW TO USE THIS BOOK

Before you dive in, I have a few comments and five key points about the material, and some tips on maximizing the application of concepts.

First, I want to be clear: The 90-Day premise of this book is only a formula for creating the foundation and suggests behavior alterations to achieve lifelong success related to fitness and nutrition. This means that you will have to work indefinitely to develop your self-love and wellness consciousness.

The reality of having to ardently apply these and other positive principles to your mindset is unavoidable should you seek sustainability. There are no short-term solutions or quick fixes, so you must passionately improve your personality and persevere. Because of this, you will notice some strategies related to attitude and awareness that easily translate to other areas of your life, not just your wellbeing.

Second, I am not a psychologist, doctor, or otherwise credentialed related to clinical behavior. My views are shaped by interacting with thousands of clients and by collecting experience. Working with and observing people, including me, struggling with fitness and nutrition sustainability, and applying common-sense solutions has been quite valuable.

The concepts in this book were developed based on that field experience, and I use real stories from actual clients to illustrate key points. I am deeply privileged to have helped thousands of people all over the world to improve their lifestyles by way of elevating personal consciousness, authenticity, and attitude towards their actions.

Third, some of the concepts you will be reading about here may seem complex, but they all tie together and are not just word salad. Buckle in, be patient with the process and fully reflect on the message if the details become overwhelming. Take time to fully process, even reread sections that seem tricky several times, and then apply. I have included chapter keynotes at the end of each chapter in Part One to assist in material comprehension and retention.

This is especially true as we explore some of my opinions related to behavior change and mindsets in Part One, such as chapters covering Wellness Consciousness, The Power of Conscious Response, Developing Intended Outcomes, and the Seven Intelligent Personality Traits. I have deliberately repeated some key concepts throughout this book to reinforce the critical nature of the subject.

Not for needless redundancy but to ensure my readers absorb the key elements through associated reinforcement and relatable stories. I should also point out that I am very direct and can sometimes write aggressively or with a touch of sarcasm to drive a concept home. I do not intend to antagonize or seem condescending to readers.

Fourth, when developing a fitness strategy, workouts, or nutrition plan, be very careful where you are getting your information. The internet is the worst place to go as there seem to be more misguided or manipulative sources than there are scientifically factual solutions. Not to worry, in Part Three of this book, we explore some scientific aspects of fitness and nutrition.

Because I did not want to make this a book full of references or unpleasant to read, all scientific claims come from the same textbooks and are referenced at the beginning of the nutrition chapter where the references are used.

Finally, if you are confused or simply don't know where to start with fitness and nutrition, I highly recommend hiring a professional coach or trainer of repute to assist you. Be certain you choose certified trainers or nutritionists that focus on systematic programming based on your unique needs.

If you are interested in working with me and my team specifically, simply visit our website at www.forgept.com and we will be happy to assist you.

PART I OVERVIEW
Habit, Behavior, and Mindset

This book is broken into three distinct parts for the consolidation of concepts and to make it easy to reference. In Part One, we will explore many of the fundamental principles of wellness consciousness, personal assessment, and means of alteration. We will review many of the challenges related to fitness and nutrition activities, and I will suggest methods to improve behavior.

This includes looking at how we interpret internal and external instigators and expose means of creating a specific personal approach to overcome undesirable negative outcomes and, instead, develop intended and positive outcomes. Again, to help with absorbing the material, at the end of all chapters in Part One I include a summary of keynotes for quick reference.

PART II OVERVIEW
90-Day Habit Transformation Workbook

This book will engage your objective personal problem solving with the application of its content. To better facilitate your efforts, I have developed and included a habit transformation workbook to support your success. This workbook serves as a guide and personal exposé to identify areas of potential improvement using techniques from Part One and further serves as a reference for future habit alteration.

PART III OVERVIEW
Sustainable Fitness and Nutrition Practices

This section eliminates all the hype, myth, or fear surrounding key fitness and nutrition principles. Taking the time to educate yourself with the truth about carbohydrates, proteins and fats will assist in creating a sustainable plan. I also outline the fundamentals of fitness programming and exercise science.

TRANSFORMATION SCHEDULE

A major stumbling block that trips most people is taking on too many complex changes all at once. We often suddenly decide we need to make a change and then get bogged down in the details and fumble along to frustration.

We get confused by conflicting information related to fitness and nutrition, so we inadvertently select convenient portions of information that suit our mindset, but this only limits our perspective and agility.

Our own bias, past success or failure, and life situations can influence how you approach improving your wellbeing. Most people rush into some convoluted diet plan or workout gimmick without addressing their root habits or considering their level of wellness consciousness.

It may seem counterintuitive, but the first steps are not necessarily choosing a diet plan or shopping, prepping, and following a strict intake. Nor is it a best practice to dive headfirst into a workout program without laying some foundation and framework from which to build.

Sustainable fitness and nutrition success comes from a strong infrastructure based on proactive habit consciousness, motivational linking, internal and external environment management, structured workouts, and a deliberate projected outcome.

We no longer have the luxury of living obliviously toward our food choices and consumption. In our modern world of unbelievably convenient access to all sorts of atrociously calorie-dense junk foods, we must be mindful of our decisions.

Another major societal issue is the overwhelming level of sedentary professions and lifestyles. This means we are likely expending far less energy than our ancestors and must be mindful of our activity as fat accumulation and postural distortions have become a growing crisis.

We need to create a mindset for identifying when we automate toward undesirable choices and have a structure in place to impede the negative habit response and provide a positive reward. Once we learn to circumvent destructive actions in our life, we can build a set of constructive actions that lead us to our intended outcome.

To do this, we need to break down the whole process into a set of weekly focus or action items. Over the years, I have developed a system for progressively improving one's mindset by methodically addressing root cause behaviors that sabotage or diminish your fitness and nutrition success. In the first week, it is critical to establish a rudimentary awareness of automated responses, choose how you will track and manage food along with planning a specialized workout program.

The first week is not supposed to be "hell week" where you find yourself frustrated with calorie counting, portion control, setting caloric goals, sorting through macro targeting, shopping, meal preparation, stressing about dining out, or a coming event. It should also not be a week where you are over-sore, working out too much or too little, doing just cardio, stressing over where to fit a workout in your schedule, and so on.

These are important details but not necessarily foundational to success when considering root habit. Yes, executing workouts and managing food will be critical for composition change and advancing wellness, but if you do not address your habits first, you are likely to cycle back into "Fitness Failure," which we cover in Part Three.

I have constructed a basic outline for the next twelve weeks and how to best apply the principles in this book. The workbook in Part Two will help you organize your approach and systematically bring attention to areas of potential improvement.

I recommend reading all of Part One of this book before filling in the workbook in Part Two. To download a full PDF version of the 90-Day Habit Transformation workbook, email us at info@forgept.com.

Week One

In this week, your objectives are to:

- Read Part One of the 90-Day Habit Transformation book.
- Evaluate your internal mindset and determine areas of consequences you would like to address immediately.
- Evaluate your external environment and determine areas of consequences you would like to address immediately.
- Set up a system for tracking your food intake. This can be intuitive, a mobile app, or traditional journaling.
- Review and understand your exercise plan and ensure it is in line with your condition and goal.
- Schedule workouts and meal preparation for the next four weeks and prioritize these activities.
- Complete the Week One activities in the 90-Day Habit Transformation Workbook.

Week Two

In this week, your objectives are to:

- Identify your Internal set of "Intrinsic Motivators" and complete the Week Two assignment in your workbook.
- Identify external or "Extrinsic Motivators" and complete the Week Two assignment in your workbook.
- Outline rewards for habit alteration or milestone successes.
- Track your food intake for each meal and snacks to create a baseline for reference and potential alteration. This should be an ongoing habit.
- Reflect on the previous week's exercises and adherence. This should be an ongoing habit.
- Complete this week's 90-Day Habit Transformation Weekly Success Journal

Week Three
In this week, your objectives are to:
- Complete your workbook assignment "Six Fitness Cornerstones of Life."
- Complete this week's 90-Day Habit Transformation Weekly Success Journal.

Week Four
In this week, your objectives are to:
- Review the last four weeks of exercise adherence and food tracking.
- Complete the "Internal and External instigator" portion of your workbook.
- Complete this week's 90-Day Habit Transformation Weekly Success Journal.

Week Five
In this week, your objectives are to:
- Complete the "Solutions Discovery" portion of the workbook.
- Outline a list of positive rewards for adhering to your plan and any rewards that need to be replaced with something proactive.
- Complete this week's 90-Day Habit Transformation Weekly Success Journal.

Week Six
In this week, your objectives are to:
- Complete the "Are You Ready to Change" portion of your workbook.
- Reflect on your position in the Stage of Change and willingness to address your discoveries made between week one and week six.
- Now that you have made significant discoveries related to motivation, the six cornerstones, your instigators, and a

set of solutions, it is time to outline a reward structure in your workbook.

- Complete this week's 90-Day Habit Transformation Weekly Success Journal.

Week Seven
In this week, your objectives are to:
- Fully commit to making change and take personal responsibility. It is time to "Clean House" by eliminating all temptations in environments you control.
- Complete the Week Seven assignment in the Workbook.
- Complete this week's 90-Day Habit Transformation Weekly Success Journal.

Week Eight
In this week, your objectives are to:
- Review the last four weeks of exercise adherence and food tracking.
- In the workbook, outline the negative effects of your most destructive habit and determine the long-term consequence. Next, define a new overwriting habit and how that will affect you immediately, and the likely long-term outcome from making that change.
- Determine your known or suspected defense mechanisms and list them in your workbook so you can be aware of potential self-sabotage and keep the Power of Conscious Response at the forefront.
- Identify and list persons who are or could be part of your support structure in your workbook.
- Complete this week's 90-Day Habit Transformation Weekly Success Journal.

Week Nine
In this week, your objectives are to:
- Based on the sum of your eight-week review, amend your action plan and develop strategies for overcoming newly discovered or lingering negative habit behaviors.
- Consider ways you can visualize the effect of negative habits and write methods of tracking or creating a visual representation of your behavior.
- Outline a habit with a monetary association and complete the exercise in your workbook for Week Nine.
- In your workbook, write your "Projected Self-Description" and "Life Quality Description."
- Complete this week's 90-Day Habit Transformation Weekly Success Journal.

Week Ten
In this week, your objectives are to:
- Take a complete look at the past ten weeks and develop a very specific plan for executing your exercises, food management, and mindset for the next 6 months. Solidify your outline and personally commit to executing the plan.
- Include others in your plan and share with at least one significant support person in your life.
- Complete this week's 90-Day Habit Transformation Weekly Success Journal.

Week Eleven
In this week, your objectives are to:
- Act on your revised plan from week ten and complete your week eleven workbook assignment by outlining long-term specifics related to how you will continue to track progress, how often you will track, and who you share this data with.
- Review your habit reward structure and make any amendments necessary to continue facilitating positive rewards for ideal behavior outcomes.

Week Twelve

In this week, your objectives are to:

- Complete the "Stress Management Strategy" portion and outline solutions for each stress type in your workbook.
- Complete this week's 90-Day Habit Transformation Weekly Success Journal.

Week Thirteen Through the Rest of Your Life

This concludes the 90-Day Habit Transformation workbook outline. Now you must focus on maintaining your life plan and execute to the best of your ability every single day. I recommend getting a fresh copy of the workbook from my website every six months to see if any instigators have diminished or changed.

Taking time to frequently reflect on your progress and keeping these concepts at the forefront of your mind will serve as an anchor. Strive not for perfection, but progress!

"

AUTHORS PERSONAL NOTE

Once I discovered that all the external pressure to meet an artificial standard was detracting from my goals and sapping joy, I learned to ignore them and work at becoming the best joyful version of me.

Chapter One
THE BEAUTY & FITNESS LIE

I would like to expose and explore several myths and societal manipulations that often negatively alter reasonable expectations and outcomes. I acknowledge I come off a bit aggressive in this chapter, but we need to be honest with ourselves and directly address these lies.

Many of these myths correlate to our desire for quick-fix solutions or to see instantaneous results with minimal effort. These issues are the direct unfavorable byproduct of a consumerist mindset and have duped people into believing they can buy fitness, beauty, or happiness.

These myths focus on superficial outcomes Instead of on creating positive and uplifting personal habits. Granted, we all want to feel beautiful, healthy, and attractive but that will require more than a crash diet, pill, or cosmetic.

Beauty is not simply an aesthetic quality; it is the collection of a persona and the quality of character we proactively develop. It is important to discuss some of these myths as many of our expectations, bias, and habits form around them.

Beauty Lies

Throughout history, the definition of beauty and the concept of fitness has constantly changed. Society, culture, economics, and technology have played a major role in how we identify and categorize aesthetic value or fitness level. It has always been subjective and before the Industrial Revolution, most of the entire world was impoverished and paid little attention to the fashions of nobility or the latest trend.

Before the nineteenth turned into the twentieth century, most people were not influenced by a mainstream media giant, nor did they possess the resources to indulge in non-essentials. Folks were too busy merely etching out the basics for survival. This has fundamentally changed, and in general, most western influenced countries enjoy remarkable abundance compared to historical counterparts.

Now add the media onslaught of mass distribution, advertising, and trends that perpetuate fabricated definitions of beauty. People around the world are buying into a superficial lie and they are loving it, or so they think. Magazines, television, movies, celebrities, and beauty companies are peddling disturbing superficial products and we just keep buying.

The frightening part of this whole mess is the age in which young people are indoctrinated into mass consumerism and superficial value systems. While many media and fitness industry players have perpetrated various lies, we will explore the top six based on what I have observed to be the most destructive.

The Skinny Lie

A dangerous and popular lie is the modern classification of skinny. Most extremes are unhealthy, and this includes underweight and overweight bodies. In general, the media defines a desirable or healthy female body as soft, curvaceous, and skinny with flawless attributes. On the other hand, men are expected to look like comic book characters with over-defined physiques and washboard abs.

This beauty ideal is largely unattainable for most, unsustainable for everyone, and has distorted the reality of what a healthy person looks like. Women of all sizes suffer the most from this unhealthy cultural direction. Most top models are not what a fitness professional would classify as healthy.

Models I have worked with are typically underweight and suffer from eating disorders and negative perceptions of the physical self. Strangely, many overweight women I have coached over the past few decades have the same problems, but without the skinny figure. This is discouraging because none of the ladies on either end of the spectrum are getting out of the media trap unscathed both psychologically and physiologically.

Sadly, this has led people to extreme actions such as cosmetic procedures including liposuction, gastric bypass, or even insulin abuse. Eating disorders such as bulimia, anorexia, binge eating, or the more recent muscle dysmorphia in men, are all products of warped body image.

No surprise, this insanity has birthed an extreme alternative mentality, which is "Your body is perfect no matter what." But folks, that is just a new lie! Your body is not "perfect" no matter what. This is a false, socially constructed bandwagon argument and a way for some people to justify an unhealthy lifestyle and absolve personal responsibility.

There is also a growing movement to simply blame one's genetics for all one's ills and lack of fitness. Again, this is a deflection of convenience because the percentage of folks whose genetic predisposition interferes with fitness or total wellbeing is extremely low compared to the general population. Yes, some genetic factors can cause health issues or challenges with composition management.

Yet the manifestation of these genetic influences can be remarkably subdued by daily activity and food management unless otherwise stated by your medical practitioner. Even if you are affected by your genes, there is no excuse for using that as a crutch and rationalization to ignore your lack of activity and reckless consumption.

That negative attitude and self-victimization only feed the genetic disposition and exacerbates the problem through low activity. Now, if you are carrying around excess body fat, regardless of if you are experiencing negative health consequences from your behavior, then you are in the same trap as an ultra-skinny person.

I understand this is a strong statement nowadays, and some become incensed by the concept of managing their problems and not blaming external factors for not "being skinny."

We largely live in a culture of hypersensitivity and disassociation from our deliberate decision-making and commit some staggering hypocritical social errors. I hear it all the time when in a social situation, particularly where food is present.

If I eat a cookie at a community event or party, someone will almost always make a comment such as "Hey, aren't you supposed to be a fitness guy? You can't eat that!"

Once, at a chamber of commerce event, this condemning cookie comment came from a person who was significantly overfat while they were shoveling a giant slice of chocolate cake into their mouth by hand. No utensils needed. I guess he thought only fat people could eat junk food. However, If I abstain from the cookie, someone will comment on my supposed obsession with fitness.

For example, later during the same chamber event, I had already abandoned my little plate and was sipping water and mingling. I was approached by a lady who asked if I was going to eat anything and before I could reply, she lectured me on not letting my obsession with fitness become a disorder. She then tried to sell me insurance. This is one example of hundreds I have experienced.

It's irritating because no matter what, someone will say something detracting. If I have a cookie on my plate, the hypocritical fitness police point it out. If no cookie is on the plate, comments are made about obsession or other such nonsense especially if people know my profession.

Many people, particularly in the media and on university campuses, love the word "shaming." I hear it used everywhere by overweight people, underweight people, and every weight between on just about any topic.

If you are fit, you get "fit-shamed," and if you are overfat, you get "fat-shamed." People can be judgmental, cynical, and jealous. If you are working toward your potential, then you have taken responsibility and may ignore all this shaming bile no matter what stage in your wellness journey you may be.

The sad point is unless we have a cultural revolution on common courtesy, these comments will affect the fit and the fat.

Social media has allowed this to become prevalent, and I point this out, so you are aware and learn to ignore it. Let me repeat that: ignore social media or any other negative comments or implications from others about your efforts to manage your lifestyle provided you are consciously seeking to improve your wellbeing. People should just keep their mouths shut and mind their own business.

As a fitness professional and courteous person, I never make commentary on others' choices unless asked directly because they want my advice or have hired me as a coach. But I don't see that decorum in most folks, especially with the prevalence of discourteous social media usage.

Anyhow, remember that the word "skinny" is a broad definition, and your genetics, body type, training style, and a whole host of factors determine your particular skinny outcome.

The Zero Blemish Lie

Cosmetics have existed for thousands of years and might be the oldest form of physical alteration to enhance appearance or desirability. However, mainstream media has bludgeoned our society to a pulp with makeup, creams, lotions, and other cosmetics. I feel there are two parts to this lie, so let's start with the obvious.

First, manufacturers and advertising agencies have set an ultra-standard of facial beauty. The models are ridiculously perfect and represent a mere fraction of a fraction of the population. And when I say "perfect," I am not advocating these models look perfect.

I am pointing out that the mainstream media is telling us that is what should be defined as perfect. The false promise is you will look the same as these genetically gifted or artificially enhanced models if you purchase and use a certain product or brand.

Second, the insinuation is that beauty is external, and these ads focus exclusively on superficial forms of beauty. Sadly, this means we often give more grace to people physically attractive from the start because the value is not in the quality of character, but aesthetics. Instagram is an incredibly potent example of beauty bias.

A dominantly nude woman doing squats will get thousands if not millions of post engagements for nothing more than showing off her body, even if her squat form is reprehensible. Compare that to an excellent instructional video for squats by a person in regular activewear showing proper form in detail. Which post do you think gets more attention?

Because of this lie, both men and women in the general population feel they should meet some impossible standard of appearance. The corrosive part is when we look in a mirror and don't see that flawless reflection of trendy beauty. This leads to potential loss of self-esteem, feelings of inadequacy, and using words like "plain" or "ugly" to describe ourselves in our head or even out loud.

Many years ago, I was training a young female athlete who was an outstanding soccer player and was remarkably fit. She was 16 years old, working for a college scholarship, and for many weeks, our sessions were positive, and she had a strong spirit. In one session, we were doing some major speed drills, cutting drills, and advanced plyometrics.

Her hair was frazzled, and her face was red from exertion, but when she noticed herself in the gym mirror, she grimaced and whispered: "God, I'm ugly." She stopped to smooth her hair, and I was heartbroken to hear how sincere her tone was and the sad look on her little face. I immediately said, "Hey, where is your head right now? Why would you say that?"

She was quiet for a moment and then just asked me point-blank, "Do you think I am ugly?" We had a good rapport, so I knew her question was innocent, but moreover, she trusted me. I simply said, "What I think, or what anyone else may think is not the right question. The real question is, why do you think you are ugly?" She replied, "I think I'm sort of ugly. I don't think I'm a troll but not as pretty as other girls." I then asked, "And just who are these girls and what about them is so beautiful?"

She listed a half-dozen celebrities and how they are always "perfect" on social media. Even more disheartening was when she showed me what she wanted to look like on some fitness models' social media pages. Each of these women she aspired to emulate promoted superficial appearance, narcissism, and perfectly posed and filtered images in exotic locations and mostly nude.

Suffice to say, I did my best to remind her of true personal beauty and encouraged her to be her own special brand of beautiful. I also told her about the lie. The nasty lies she believed enough to even think for a moment she was ugly. I suspect that my brief chat with her was not enough to overcome the daily avalanche of social media influence.

We all go through periods of self-doubt or feelings of inadequacy, but this was beyond that. This was from a 16-year-old athlete in peak physical condition with a potential D1 scholarship, excellent grades, and a very pretty look, but she defined beauty just as the media programmed: unobtainable, unsustainable, and superficial.

The Fashion Lie

As much as I enjoyed the film "The Devil Wears Prada," I find some components of fashion to be truly silly. There is little value in mainstream fashion as far as I am concerned, but I know many people who find aspects of fashion a form of artistic expression and function. Fine.

I understand that part, but there are some strong ethical issues surrounding fashion. Most notorious is the body image influence we already explored. But the fashion industry has done more than just lie to us about beauty and social acceptance; they have virtually altered human physiology. For fashion, technology is a powerful tool to propagate their fabrication and cultural manipulation.

Computer programs have allowed for excessive and inappropriate augmentation of skin texture and body shape. They take genetically gifted men and women with unusually well-proportioned parts and then create a whole new false species of human that not one of us will ever look like in our lifetimes.

I find this remarkably disturbing and imagine the cover model they altered looking in the mirror to see a body that is not the same as the one on the magazine cover and having to reconcile that emotionally.

What must he or she think of themselves when they are in bad dressing room lighting and there is little similarity between their cover photo and real life? No wonder we have eating disorders, body issues, and psychological problems running rampant in the fashion model profession.

Of course, this series of destructive behaviors have saturated the public as well. The fashion lie includes the claim that what you bought last season is no longer fashionable, which is to say you are no longer trendy or beautiful. I acknowledge there are many layers to the fashion industry, but our focus is on the manipulation of the beauty perspective.

How often have you been in a social situation where someone negatively remarked on your sweater, dress, shoes, jeans, or accessories? There you are, enjoying lunch with a group of friends when one of them titters at you with "Oh, is that the last season Louie? Well, mine is the latest from Paris and I simply love-love-love it."

Or you are a man in an office and a coworker snicker at you "Soooo, pleated pants? Did you raid your grandpa's dresser to dig those up? Lol, It's all about the flat front now." This mentality is shallow and discourteous and another good example of when people should reconsider their comments.

However, sometimes people do dress awkwardly or mismatched to the point of distracting or inappropriate for the situation. This is separate from fashion shaming or implying someone is not attractive.

Fitness Lies

I hope that discussing these topics will bring awareness and objectivity to each of you regarding the media and how we respond as consumers. Unfortunately, the fitness industry has expanded on some of the beauty lies by creating their own fancy set. I find it shameful how the fitness industry, which purports a healthy lifestyle, subscribes to unhealthy behaviors.

If you skipped the earlier chapter on How I Shaped My Philosophy, go back and read it for my full opinion on the fitness industry in general. The exploitation and manipulation of people's emotional frailty regarding beauty and fitness are irresponsible, and so many fitness institutions are guilty. I have narrowed down my opinion on the top three most insidious lies in the fitness industry.

The Gimmick Lie

Starting with the gimmick lie sets the foundation for the other two fitness lies. As a fitness professional, I get very frustrated with the endless production and reproduction of useless products pumped out by the mainstream fitness industry. Mainly because gimmick products will not work, and this places people back into the cycle of fitness failure, which is the perpetual succession of starting a program or diet that deteriorates into another failed attempt to meet a fitness or health goal.

Repeated failure only breeds discouragement, declined self-esteem and eventually, you will just submit to the condition. For this segment, I focused more on wide main-stream-media based gimmicks and not so much on gyms themselves. Anyway, let's explore some mainstream gimmick examples.

The most obvious are weights that shake, wearable saunas, things that slide, glide or rock. Belts that vibrate, blades that wobble, topical products, or anything with the word "tone" in it. But the mainstream media is clever and recognizes that the market is more informed than ever. And because many of us have been swindled in the past, we have become more skeptical of products and services and like to research and validate before we buy.

To combat our new resistance, the media machine will use "science" and "doctors' to endorse products. With this false credibility, they pulled one over on us again. We fall for it every time! Now we have fake science and sell-out doctors leading the charge against the consumer pushing a new line of gimmicks. And to be frank, the biggest scam in the fitness industry is the diet pill.

Two problems with diet pills and supplements. First, what is in the pill or supplement, and how do we verify that the content, quality, and advertised effects are genuine? We don't and we can't.

The supplement industry is not regulated by any form of quality assurance. This means they can sell you a 5,000-milligram pill where 3,500 milligrams are classified as "proprietary blend," and you can't even pronounce the top five ingredients they do list other than caffeine, niacin, or another base mineral.

The return on investment for supplementation is negligible for most people who are not bodybuilders or avid exercisers. Meaning there are supplements out there that provide some benefits but it's usually specialized. Yet, the gimmick industry alone pulls in billions of dollars because of the second problem: We keep buying it.

But why? Exercise, moderating diet, and managing our general fitness can be hard and it requires new habits, perseverance, and maintenance. We even have planned excuses ready to exonerate our latest failed attempt at a diet or workout. I hear them daily, such as family, time, money, energy, or career, but this is how we self-justify our behavior.

Folks, there is no quick fix or magic pill to improve composition, endurance, or strength. You must put in the effort and change your behavior. And you must ignore what other people look like or what the media is saying you should look like. Just be the very best version of yourself.

The Nutrition Lie

Nutrition in America today has become cult-like with its own dogma. Before the mini-apocalypse of 2020, conversations about politics inspired less hostility than a vegan vs keto advocate debating. It's obnoxious and unnecessary. The media has done a fantastic job of spinning false information or manipulated data about macronutrient food quality and appropriate intake ratios to sell products.

If you think that industrial farms for livestock, dairy, or plant products are not lobbying both government and media to validate their goods for profit, then you are missing out. However, addressing all the issues surrounding nutrition, misinformation, and mega-food corporation influence is not within the scope of this book, but we need to acknowledge it.

The science of nutrition is so complex, and the media has simplified it to the point of ineffectual. As a former college instructor of advanced health and fitness sciences, I taught two nutrition classes. The first was basic college nutrition and the second was nutrition for sports performance, and I still learn new things or paradoxes about nutrition all the time.

I hold two nutrition-based credentials, one for the science of nutrition and one for nutrition-based life coaching, and they are a drop in the ocean of nutritional studies. Even a basic college textbook for first-semester nutrition only scratches the surface. Dietitians and professors of nutritional studies are still making discoveries in this field.

There is no one-size-fits-all diet plan and very few nutritional experts. However, many people have tried with fanatical zeal, a diet that is either fat-free, high fat, low-carb, low-sugar, high-fiber, high-protein, grain-free, vegan, vegetarian, pescatarian, plant-based, no fruit, only fruit, no legumes, no dairy, macro-focused, volumetric, raw-only, macrobiotic, blood type based, intermittent fasting, gluten-free, juicing, carnivorous and ketogenic diets.

Yup, that was a run-on sentence to illustrate the insanity and saturation of all this nutrition nonsense. Each of these fad diets has the same formula: elimination of food types, reduction of a macro, and restriction of calories. Let me clarify: What makes a fad diet different from another fad diet, is simply what macro or food sources you eliminate or reduce with calorie restriction.

It's so challenging to cut through the mainstream media hype or their rabid focus on a specific component of nutrition. I remember in the 1990s the demonization of fat and the emergence of the green label and reduced-fat foods, which gave way to the ultra-high protein diet, but that's unsustainable and gone.

Then a celebrity, who truly has a verified and diagnosed medical condition, starts talking about gluten, writes a book, and the media sees a profit center. We are still suffering to this day from consumer overreaction and mass self-diagnose of gluten intolerance.

This excludes those of you with serious conditions such as Celiac, Crohn's, Candida, or any other official medical diagnosis. But that fad is fading now because suddenly we are on a trip back through time to prehistoric food selection.

Except for most foods we have today would not have been available to our ancestors, but hey, it's a good gimmick and folks fall for it. What about the wildly popular epileptics diet, also known as ketogenic. The common theme here is a desperate consumer seeking a solution and unable to sort through the myths, misinformation, and manipulated data designed to sell products.

On the other hand, the mainstream media only advertise what sells. Every famous gimmick or diet out there is a byproduct of consumer demand. The media knows we want products that claim to work quickly, require little or no effort, and are stylish. We can stop the spread of silly diets and useless products by simply not buying them. We are all at fault as media is the product of our design.

So, unless you are on a medically supervised nutritional program for a specific condition, here is my opinion: Your nutritional intake or "diet" should be nutrient-dense, calorically appropriate for fitness goals, and consisting of loose macro ratios you can sustain for a lifetime. This means that if a configuration of nutrition and calories meets the requirements of your lifestyle and wellness goal, then you have found your diet.

The Duration Lie

This lie is a major source of irritation for me and fitness professionals around the world. The duration lie is the time in which the mainstream fitness media claims their product or service will profoundly change your fitness level or life. Duration has become a shining beacon of consumer gullibility and growing societal desire for instant gratification, plus this lie antagonizes my dislike for devious marketing.

The fitness industry is inundated by gimmicks as we discussed and now, we have 8-minute abs, 4, 6, and 12-week challenges where you get duped into believing you can look like a fitness model just by following some generic workout template you bought off a genetically gifted professional exerciser on Instagram.

These so-called "influencers" are paid by corporations to promote their products or apparel and are rarely even certified trainers. They just get paid to work out and look as good as possible to sell you stuff or fuel their OnlyFans subscriptions.

They also make bold statements about losing large amounts of fat in extremely narrow periods and usually forcefully recommend buying their sponsored supplement as well.

This is predatory marketing and a flat-out lie. Any generic program that promises highly specific returns is questionable because each human has a unique fitness level, medical condition, injury history, nutritional sensitivity, schedule, resource access, and desire.

I also find before-and-after pictures of others to be manipulative marketing and an extremely unhealthy reason to join a program, especially if accompanied by an advertised time frame in which those results were supposedly achieved.

That is why I do not post before and after photos on my website. These success stories are not yours, nor is that before-and-after body yours. We should focus on our before-and-after pictures and celebrate our fitness progressions. This leads me to my point, on how human physiology changes with stress and is a key component to estimating how long it may take to achieve a particular goal.

The Principle of Specificity indicates the human body will specifically adapt to an imposed demand. Meaning for example, that if you apply resistance to the bicep in a curl with 10 lbs under certain acute variables, then the body will make biomechanical and neuromuscular adaptations to meet the demand.

Initially, the 10 lbs may be challenging but over a period called a mezzo cycle, the body adapts and 10 lbs is no longer the same challenge. You must then change the acute variables to inspire further adaptation.

The time it takes to go from struggling to lift the 10 lbs to meeting the challenge is quite predictable provided the proper acute variables are followed and this allows a competent person to estimate return over time.

Just to clarify, acute variables in exercise program design include load, sets, repetitions and contraction tempo, training intensity, training volume, rest interval, exercise selection, exercise order, training duration, and training frequency.

Yes, some people follow a crash course diet and fitness program and shed large amounts of weight. I have seen people lose four to five pounds in a week, but it is nearly always temporary. These people are usually very overweight individuals whose bodies are begging to lose the excess. And, often, they are in a state of deprivation such as starvation or some other form of eating and exercise disorder.

Not what I call the picture of health and sustainability. How many people do you know that lost significant weight in some program just to gain it all back plus some? It happens all the time. It's called fitness failure and people are stuck in this hopeless cycle. But this happens because people don't think about the whole process.

You don't gain 50 lbs of body fat in 12 weeks. It takes months or even years to accumulate in a general adult. What makes us think it's possible to lose that amount in 12 weeks? But the mainstream media will prey on your desire for instant reward and results. So, you try another program and for the first few days or weeks, you are all in and committed until it gets hard, or you see no immediate transformation.

The media is lying not only about the time it will take to regain control of your body, but you want to believe the lie. It's easy, convenient, and makes you feel like you're finally doing something. But what you likely get are feelings of regret and backsliding.

And just like every time before, you soon give up until the next shiny gimmick comes along and snares you again. You can purchase 100% of a program but if you don't do the work, your results are highly predictable as zero.

Acknowledge that maintaining your body, the vessel of your mind and soul will require effort and commitment. I challenge you to cast aside the fads and gimmicks and find a fitness program that supports you and your unique situation. Something you can make part of your life and sustain indefinitely. But first, you must change your habits.

A Note on The Body Positive Movement

I feel taking a moment to express my view on all types or forms of body positivity movements is an important capstone to this chapter. I want to be crystal clear, people should never be judged or criticized based on their regular appearance, size, weight, gender, race, ethnicity, and so on.

It's mostly none of our business how people choose to live or how they treat their bodies. While it can be startling or sad to see self-abuse and neglect, we typically do not have the whole story and should withhold judgment.

However, there is a big difference between finding self-love where we truly and deeply love ourselves versus abusing our bodies and using a social crutch to justify our destructive choices or behavior. Yes, I agree our society can be superficial and mean-spirited, especially on social media.

Yet we must be constantly working to become the best version of ourselves. We are all at different stages in our life and elevating our consciousness toward wellbeing. But abusing one's body with excessive eating and obesity is just as destructive as any eating disorder.

I think learning to love the nuances of our bodies is a remarkably empowering mindset and I strongly encourage this.

This includes the appreciation and acceptance of our genetic disposition but in the context of being reasonably fit and not using excuses for our condition.

There are some things out of our control, but we must overcome these situations or limitations each day to continue growing and finding our joy. I strongly encourage folks to not use a social movement as a shield or justification for poor food choices or laziness but appreciate the spirit of the movement towards self-love.

Chapter Keynotes

The primary intention of this chapter is to help readers set aside unrealistic and socially constructed expectations of beauty and fitness. We need to focus on becoming the best we can as individuals and ignore the media definition of beauty or fitness. Here are some bullet points for quick reference:

- Many of these myths correlate to our desire for quick-fix solutions or to see instantaneous results with minimal effort.
- It is important to address some of these myths as many of our expectations, bias, and habits form around them.
- Society, culture, economics, and technology have played a major role in how we identify and categorize aesthetic value or fitness level.
- Magazines, television, movies, celebrities, and beauty companies are peddling superficial products and we keep buying despite the consequences.
- We should focus on our before-and-after pictures and celebrate our personal fitness progressions.
- There is a big difference between finding self-love where we truly and deeply love ourselves versus abusing our bodies and using a social crutch to justify our destructive choices or behavior.
- Compare yourself to yourself and work to be the absolute best version of yourself.
- I strongly encourage folks to not use a social movement as a shield or justification for poor food choices or laziness but appreciate the spirit of the body positive movement towards self-love.

Habit alteration is a slow process and quitting won't speed it up.

Chapter Two
THE BASICS OF HABIT

I define habits as an acquired set of behaviors that have become almost involuntary, rooted deep in our subconscious through patterns and instigated responses. These learned responses are reinforced by repetition and the more powerful habits are often accompanied by an emotional trigger, which I call an instigator.

As an arching theme, habit tendencies are usually linked to the avoidance of pain or pursuing pleasure. Habits result from efficiency adaptations, but for our purposes, we will focus more on the instigators, actions, and rewards toward fitness and nutrition. Generalized habits alone are not good or bad, but the nature of the habit can be classified based on your relationship with the activity.

For example, the habit of brushing one's teeth is positive and the benefits are unquestionable. However, fanatic or obsessive brushing and flossing can cause damage to tooth enamel and gums. The habit of binge eating after a stressful day is certainly not healthy behavior, but a balanced and nutrient-dense food intake is.

We can cite hundreds of examples where a regular activity can become an instigator or obsession forming a negative habit. Developing habits and the repetitive execution of behavior or autonomous acts are only the beginning. There must be some sort of reward driving the actions, but they are only the result of an internal or external instigator. In a later chapter, I dive deeply into a concept called the "Power of Conscious Response" but want to make a few notes about habit before we get to that part.

Habits Are Efficiency Adaptations

Habits create continuity, efficiencies, and reward in our daily activities. The automation of response is a necessary component of human function as not every single decision can be made intentionally. Therefore, we must be proactive in our formation of habits, especially those with consequences, and prioritize our efforts there.

Diverting energies to affect personal change based on your projected outcome will be critical for success. Yet, it would be impossible to try and stop every moment in time or interrupt interactions so you can deliberate on a course of action or respond. Our minds want to formulate efficiencies just like our bodies. In exercise physiology, we call this the General Adaptation Syndrome theory tied to periodization.

Essentially, with stress or repetition, the biomechanical and neuromuscular aspects of the human body create efficiency adaptations to accommodate a specific demand allowing for higher levels of performance. However, adaptation efficiencies in your body are not always positive, just like habit efficiencies are not always positive.

To clarify, in exercise physiology, adaptations can serve to positively increase mobility, neuromuscular coordination, endurance, and strength. Yet, negative adaptations from a sedentary lifestyle may cause mobility issues, joint malalignment, decreased performance, or strength. In the formation of habit efficiencies, progress would be considered a positive habit, while a regression would be a negative habit.

In exercise, you have plateaus, overtraining, and undertraining, but the principle of efficiency is the same so that's why I compare them because you must be consciously proactive and apply the proper stresses to elicit the desired result.

As I stated earlier, with positive wellness-based habit formation, we must apply a deliberate set of actions based on a known instigator, a planned response, and a reward aligned with our outcome objective.

We can't be a passenger on this ride and must be completely engaged in our conscious response related to areas we want to improve.

Therefore, it is so important we take time to identify those negative or destructive habits that are automated and pay them special attention for alteration. Otherwise, we just get stuck in an automated and destructive response cycle.

Habit and Resistance - Oscillation

We will resist changing or adding a new habit for several reasons. Even though we all know change is inevitable, we resist because it pulls us out of homeostasis, removes predictability, and instigates the fear of loss. Let's talk about homeostasis first, as that is one of the more interesting aspects in my estimation because it affects many of our internal systems.

Homeostasis is simply a state of stability physically, mentally, and environmentally. The biggest homeostatic conflict I see with my new clients and most people starting a fitness program is oscillation. It is essentially a massive overcorrection, which leads to negative feedback and regression. The most common example is that of the crash or fad dieter.

For a few years now, I have worked with a young lady who used to go through periods of oscillation based on what she saw on social media. While her tendency to suddenly want to uproot her entire training approach and food program has diminished greatly, it is still something she must be conscious of.

When we first met, she was just coming out of a several-month stint with what looked like some kind of odd Paleo diet mashup having just spent the past three months before that on a restrictive ultra-low-fat diet where she eliminated nearly all fat other than fish.

No nuts, no grains, no legumes, no seeds, no oils, no red meats, no poultry, no eggs or avocado. From a dietary standpoint, this is the total opposite in food choice reversal in less than 6 months.

She had an estimated sedentary output of approximately 1,900 calories and was taking in about 800-1,000 and that was about the same consumption on both the super low-fat diet and then the Paleo approach. During the time she was on the low-fat diet, she was also doing an extremely aggressive and popular Olympic lift style workout 3-4 days each week, so her probable output was near the 2,300-2,600 mark.

Like most people not properly conditioned for this trendy workout style, she inevitably got injured and decreased her activity. In her convalescence, she followed a social media "influencer" who was a professional exerciser and advertiser all about Paleo and those ridiculous "booty band" workouts.

You know, the ones where they focus almost exclusively on building the butt and do a half-billion squats and lunges, step-ups, and so on with an excessive arch in the low back to make sure it's worthy of Instagram to get as much attention as possible.

So, she ditched the aggressive workout style and the low-fat diet and went all-in on the booty workouts and a loose Paleo diet. Anyhow, over the six months, you can see she went from one extreme to another, but her composition barely changed at all.

The only success she was having was making herself miserable, resenting fitness, and inevitably just crashing on her diet. She would gain weight, freak out, and overreact to a new fad program. Same formula as every fad, which is caloric restriction, demonization of a macro, and overemphasis on a single food source.

I spent several weeks having to build trust with her because she expected to jump into another fad diet and wanted instant results. The problem was we did not have a proper baseline to work with, and her impatience was circumventing the usual application of moderation and consistency in program design and nutritional intake.

I suggested we just hit the reset button and trust the process. She had nothing to lose and after some gentle mindset coaching, she found balance. I started her with a simple calorically appropriate and nutritionally dense set of menu suggestions approximately 1,400-1,500 calories, with around 40% from complex carbohydrates, 30% protein, and 30% fats.

I also built her a structured fitness program that was periodized so we could validate the results and systematically apply stressors to elicit a predictable outcome. Of course, she melted down at the idea of eating over 1,000 calories and not switching her workouts each week. She had been thoroughly brainwashed by the media and irresponsible social media trainers peddling garbage preying on the fears and hopes of the vulnerable.

More than that, she had never built healthy habits based on discipline, she did it out of a short-term obsession. We will cover obsession versus discipline in a later chapter, but my point is, she had oscillated so often she had never really formed any constructive habits. What she did was create an unhealthy relationship with food and grew to despise exercise.

On top of all that, she feared change. Her homeostasis was oscillating and causing her to slow the distance that the pendulum swung caused fear. If the programs were not extreme, her mind could not reconcile potential effectiveness. She thought nutrition was about starving all day and workouts were supposed to be painful.

On the bright side, the proper application of exercise and responsible energy intake resulted in her finally dropping body fat by several percentage points in just a few months. Her lean tissue went from 72 lbs to nearly 77 lbs in about four months. She still has tendencies to come to a coaching call questioning nearly every aspect of a new workout plan, but that's also part of her personality.

Habit and Resistance – Selective Knowledge

Very few people enjoy looking foolish or feeling ignorant. It is why we fear public speaking, the first day of school, or dating, for example. In fitness, the lack of knowledge ties into the fear of failure we will explore soon, but we will look at how too much or a lack of knowledge can create habit resistance.

I see this in two forms, the first is arrogance or subscription to dogma where people research, compare, and digest as much information about their choice as possible. These people are looking to validate their decisions, ensure they have a structure and there are aspects of tribalism present in most cases.

The second resistance is ignorance, confusion from conflicting information or not understanding what approach is best for oneself. These folks do not understand where to start, what to eat, how to exercise, or manage their wellbeing. In both cases, we see a selective application of knowledge, which is a form of resistance.

In the first scenario of the arrogantly educated, many people can get tied up in a specific kind of workout or diet plan and become unwilling to explore alternatives. This is the case even if the subscribed approach is no longer or has never even worked, which baffles me. I see this very frequently with diets, but it happens with fitness modalities as well.

Supposed knowledge becomes a resistance when we are comfortable, or our peer group is involved so we don't have to think. Tribalism is often key here, as seen in just about every popular workout style or fad diet. The media also plays a big role, especially with hyper-popularized fads. "If these many people are doing it, it must work, right?" Wrong, that's another bandwagon fallacy.

But we become emotionally connected to specific approaches and resist change even if what may have been effective for a period, is now producing little or no return. For example, The Keto diet was awesome initially and you lost all this weight, which was cool and that reinforced your subscription to the approach. Then over time, you find this diet is unsustainable for you, so your results and adherence wanes.

Where oscillation is not the response, we cling to many aspects of what worked in the past. I have been working with a young woman for many years and when we first met, she was a Keto disciple.

Her results had waivered significantly, and with her schedule, she could not maintain the preparation and focus to remain in ketosis. But she was ultra-resistant to any other food lifestyle and over the first few months, she kept trying to incorporate Keto although it was not reasonable.

On top of this, she had a specific vegetarian diet as well. No gluten, no grains, no meats of any kind, and restrictive. Her intake rarely exceeded 1,000 calories and vegetarian Keto menus are extremely difficult to adhere to because as a plant-based eater your carb intake will naturally be over twenty-five grams in most cases. She was a restaurant server by day, barkeeping by night, and exercised four to five times each week but inconsistently.

Her average output was nearly 2,100-2,300 calories each day. Her workouts were not very intense, she was always fatigued, and she resented her fitness and food lifestyle.

It took months of coaching, but finally, she relented and moved to a more balanced and reasonable lifestyle and was able to manage a vegetarian intake. We altered her from five workouts each week to only three with the intention of higher intensity and focus.

Her caloric intake was increased to 1,900 with an average deficit of about 250-500 calories, so she experienced less fatigue and all but lost the desire to binge late at night. She was doing great for nearly a year and then decided she wanted to try Keto again.

She felt there were inherent health benefits to it based on her previous bias and her ongoing YouTube education. Now that her body composition was where she wanted it, she returned to her failed belief system. Fine. I helped her transition smoothly and within two months, she hit a wall and regressed.

Although Keto was her dogmatic preference, she could not even make it work in her life. She would go through cycles of resistance and regressions. This is a self-imposed problem and being flexible in your approach allows for a higher level of satisfaction and consistency without the cycling failures.

She has recently reembraced the reasonable vegetarian lifestyle she can manage and has abandoned the Keto approach. She is doing great again.

In our second scenario of selective knowledge, we have beginners or people who have extraordinarily little functional knowledge about fitness or nutrition.

Lack of knowledge creates resistance because people fear injury, poor results, judgment, disruption to comfort, and recognizing they must put forth a good deal of effort to improve. Learning something new, especially if you don't want to, can be a powerful resistance to change.

This group is particularly susceptible to latching onto small pieces of information and forming an unfounded resistance. I have a rare but interesting case example. One of my long-time clients with whom I work on mindset coaching and advanced fitness likes to supplement our work together with a small group, High-Intensity Interval Training class.

Well, my client had referred one of her very overweight co-workers who was less than a novice in fitness and nutrition. My client explained to her how she meets with me every other week on video chat and the level of detail we developed for her fitness programming and nutrition coaching. She also explained she supplements with the live group class twice each week.

However, her co-worker did not want to attend a live class because of her extremely deconditioned state. Yet she selectively heard and held onto the notion of HIIT training and believed it was the right way to work out and anything else was wrong or a waste of time. But her medical situation, condition level, joint health, and proprioceptive response were very debilitated.

This situation is grounds to avoid aggressive exercise, jumping, and movements like burpees because they are not the correct application of stress. She was well over 280 lbs with acquired diabetes and had never formally exercised in her life. I explained to her that based on her condition, we would need to start with fundamentals focused on mobility, joint integrity, and progressive application of stress to ramp up to HIIT.

Despite my experience and knowledge, she clung to the idea of HIIT because of my other client's success and what she read about HIIT online. She was not sincerely looking to make a habitual change; she was looking for a quick fix and thought HIIT would be the answer.

Over a few sessions, I worked to gain rapport and trust to overcome resistance so I could outline a progressive plan that moved her from the habits that got her to the condition she was in. I showed her how to understand nutritional basics and prudently incorporate appropriate exercise structures. I use her as an example because, from the very beginning, she had unusual resistance.

Essentially, I discovered she was trying to find a way to eat candy bars, ice cream, and pizzas without changing habits or exercising consistently. She thought that if she worked out hard a few times, restricted calories, or followed macros, she could eat anything she wanted.

Her lack of knowledge became a resistance because she did not seek to learn but instead would find snippets of selective information that supported her poor food choices. Thus, a lack of knowledge can be deliberate. On the bright side, those people who are serious about improving become less resistant to altering their habits.

Results inevitably follow once they open their minds, learn what works for them and eliminate resistance. But it is a decision one must make and commit to. She never did and has since returned to her sedentary and destructive lifestyle.

Habit and Resistance – Return Versus Effort

Of all the habit resistances, return versus effort is the most cynical and surprisingly common. Essentially, this is when we resist making change because we fear the effort will be greater than our perceived return. It is also sometimes tied to the fear of disruption and the fear of exhaustion. When we evaluate our lifestyle and any changes to it, we generally act in pursuing pleasure or the avoidance of pain. Ironically, resistance in this form only delays return even further. You get nothing for nothing.

The comfort of predictability and pain we already know can sabotage the development of healthy habits. We settle for the familiar pain instead of the potential unknown pain of change. Often, people who resist in this manner have experienced repeated failed attempts to alter their habits or wellness. They know how hard it was last time and the results were not commensurate with their effort.

Yet when we examine these cases, we find that the attempt was almost always through a gimmick, fad diet, or incorrect exercise approach. Another observation is that people jump on programs with a specified timeline and never actually change root habits to accommodate a lifestyle. Like I said earlier, your efforts must exceed the 90 days of institutional change outlined within this book.

The good news is lack of knowledge and misdirection of energy is a problem we can solve. I have two examples to share with you related to the resistance of return versus effort. First, I have worked with a young lady for quite some time and this resistance is her primary roadblock. She is well organized and has all aspects of her wellness needs aligned. She has meals delivered to her, a gym in her community complex, and a gym at work.

She meets with me every single week and has the support of her husband and teenage son. She has her workouts scheduled for five days each week and they are built specifically to her needs. The problem is, she comes to her coaching calls with less than a quarter of her workouts completed nearly every week. Why? Everything is set and all she must do is execute her workouts.

She is resisting because she is afraid that if she does the workouts, she will not see a substantial return and it will not be worth it to spend the energy. I recently said to her, "Well, you are getting the same outcome you are trying to avoid by not doing the work." That seemed to resonate, and she began to slowly improve her exercise adherence. She has nothing to lose by just doing her workouts. They are only 45 minutes and when she does them, she always reports feeling better.

Granted, she has her nutrition dialed and has significantly improved her mindset and lifestyle in general. Yet she was not achieving her potential because she avoided activity. The funny thing is, when I wrote this, it has been five weeks of her hitting every workout and she has reduced her body fat by over one percent, which relates to just around three pounds of pure fat for her. Imagine where she would be now if she did not resist when she started nine months ago.

The second example is on the extreme side, and I only encounter this intensity of resistance infrequently, but I feel it's worth examining. I worked with a woman for about three months who resisted everything. I don't think I am exaggerating much when I say "everything" either. She refused to workout, refused to track her food for any period, refused to clean the house and manage her environment, and avoided any self-reflection.

Meaning when I had her do the weekly homework in the 90-day workbook, it was incomplete or not done at all. She was very pleasant, and we had nice conversations and rapport, but she simply resisted everything in polite defiance.

I wanted to understand her inability to simply make some small alterations to achieve the very purpose for which she hired me. After one of our last coaching calls, she revealed that because she was so intensely obese and deconditioned, she felt it would be too hard to ever get well, so why bother.

She had crossed over so far that she believed the effort was not worth all the rewards of fitness. She had tried so often over twenty years to correct her life path, but she was so ingrained and comfortable with her pain that the anticipated new and unknown pain of change would be too much. She also tried to buy her fitness.

She enrolled in a major coaching or clinical program every few years and her history was to quit or not adhere. She spent thousands and thousands of dollars on programs over the years and never followed through. This is because the act of purchasing a program gave her just a moment of gratification and hope, but when it came time for the work, she was not truly ready to change. She had a deep set of limiting beliefs and in the stages of change, she never got past the Preparation phase, which we will review the chapter after next.

Habit and Resistance – Fear

Fear of change can be quite subtle and elusive from your conscious realization on the one hand or be obvious and identifiable on the other. The level of fear and associated resistance varies from person to person, but we all feel it. Fear-born anxiety is double-edged because it can inspire action or cause paralysis, so it is important to courageously meet fears head-on and address the source of your resistance and act.

Let's address some common fear-based resistances such as disruption of homeostatic routine, fear of failure, fear of guilt, and fear of exhaustion.

Fear of Disruption

Disruption of homeostatic routine is simply the fear of having your comfort zone or habits challenged. It's fascinating that even our negative routines that have greatly influenced our discontented state can impede our desire to make a change. We must eliminate the fear of disruption by addressing solutions that will resolve the negative consequences of our behavior. When we are comfortable, we often become complacent. Let's look at an example of how to positively disrupt destructive habits based on the comfort of routine.

I work with a gentleman who has spent several years in the relative comfort of predictability but had suffered significant health-related issues because of the level of destructive homeostatic comfort. He contacted me to help him make a change and overcome the fear because he was finding the quality of his life was deteriorating in several areas and his homeostatic routine was a major factor. He is a traveling salesperson on the road about every other week or so and the nature of his profession requires a good deal of sitting in meetings, dining with clients, and long hours.

In his spare time, he would play online video games or binge-watch television shows compounding the negative effects of a low activity level profession, with a sedentary personal lifestyle. The fear of changing his routine was double-pronged because he could not see a solution to meetings or long hours. He also contributed much of his professional success to his dinner and cocktail meetings and was afraid to change his sales and client retention approach because he felt these interactions were a primary reason for his rapport and later success with clients.

On the other prong, he found levity and escape from the rigors of his job by playing video games with a group of other gamers. His television shows also allowed him to disconnect. In our coaching sessions, we created a more inclusive mindset related to his work, hobbies, and wellness. I like to work backward by identifying how aspects of one's life improve with higher levels of fitness, nutrition management, and overall sense of wellbeing.

We often attempt to compartmentalize fitness in one box, nutrition in another, and then further separate work from personal life. This is an unrealistic approach, and we must strive to make our lives more inclusive, which I will explore in the later chapter. Once we agree that all aspects of our lives cannot effectively be rigidly compartmentalized or quarantined, we can work to create positive inclusivity.

In my example case, we had to ratify why his fitness and food choices were important and how to make this inclusive. We came up with several strategies for his client's meal and cocktail hours by improving food choice, serving size, and volume of drinking. This allowed him to make better choices within the conditions of his work life, which ultimately translated to his personal life.

As a side note, when he and his partner would go to dinner, he automatically made better choices without sacrificing the value of dining out and sharing time with his significant other. He overcame his fear of damaging his career by simply changing his self-imposed rules to be in line with his wellness goals. He did not need to sacrifice his professional approach, but his initial fear did not allow him to consider any alternatives or see the solution was quite simple.

Now, we had to address his sedentary personal lifestyle and the poor food choices made from convenience. This was more difficult because he did not want to eliminate his time spent with video games. No problem. We agreed that he would do a 30-minute workout before gaming and instead of ordering pizza, which was his routine, he would have a nutritious meal prepared. We eliminated the negative consequences of making a poor food choice of convenience by having a healthy alternative.

He did not have to sacrifice gaming and he made a once-a-week allowance for sharing a small pizza with his partner provided he did a full hour workout beforehand. The half pizza was also contingent on a commitment he did at least four of his scheduled five workouts that week despite how busy things got. He also limited his television viewing significantly and used that time to exercise instead. By applying inclusive principles, setting boundaries, and making minor alterations to his choices he maintained the areas of his life he most valued.

He still wines and dines clients and prospects, plays video games, eats pizza occasionally, and has developed healthy personal boundaries. He has gone from a completely sedentary life void of exercise to consistently exercising well over five days each week. He has fundamentally transformed his attitude toward fitness and nutrition and incorporates wellness into his general mindset. He has turned his negative homeostatic routine into a positive homeostatic routine, which provides that comfort of predictability without damage.

His body composition has greatly improved as well and his lean muscle, endurance, and strength have all increased. His total body fat has dropped significantly showing more definition than ever in his adult life.

Fear of Failure

Fear is a paralyzing agent in fitness and nutrition lifestyle management for several reasons. First, we fear we are choosing the wrong fitness activity or diet plans. We become so inundated with contradictory information that we fear choosing the wrong path and wasting time, money, motivation, and not seeing progress. Second, procrastination is a common problem we must overcome to maintain our focused workouts and discipline around food choices.

The procrastination just reinforces the fears, and we justify why we can't seem to make it work. It's quite a vicious cycle and can be hard to break unless you are applying the Power of Conscious Response and setting reasonable goals for yourself. Another paralyzer is the fear of not being fit enough to start a workout plan or go to the gym in general. We fear we may be judged or look foolish trying to figure out a machine and perhaps perform exercises incorrectly.

Many people fear over-soreness or exacerbating an old injury so it's easy to avoid even starting. I have even heard people say they want to wait to hire a trainer until after they get back in shape. This makes no sense at all and is just another form of fear manifesting procrastination. My experience has shown me the excuse of not hiring a professional until you are in better shape is usually the fear of wasting money. We doom our wellness journey from the beginning because we have experienced so much fitness failure in the past, it is now our expected outcome.

I will cover fitness failure later but suffice to say, it is the common outcome for most Americans. I am sure some people may feel embarrassed about their condition and suspect a trainer would be judgmental, so they avoid it. I have seen foolish trainers use belittlement or other divisive approaches thinking they are motivating, but this is a terrible coaching technique. Sadly, some celebrity trainers made themselves famous and built whole brands by yelling at clients, which has been popular on national reality television. This is an appalling practice in real life and is a false representation of most fitness professionals.

Finally, fear can be completely counterintuitive and when tied to extremes, produce a strong resistance. Most people are attached to an approach and have a very hard time detaching even though it is not working. They fear the change will make things worse and so doggedly cling to the mast of a sinking ship. Don't be afraid to fail because it's not about whether you fail, it's about whether you keep trying.

One of the most common I experience is in young women. Imagine a woman who is between 5' 10" and 6' who at one point ate 800-1,000 calories each day as a teenager and young adult while exercising several times each week but not necessarily in a structured manner. The grace of youth forgives many mistakes, but as she ages, her metabolic and hormonal responses can change significantly.

Now this woman is in her early 30s and noticing a decrease in her performance and her body composition. She becomes soft and her figure becomes less defined and finds herself getting ill or injured often. Let's say her exercise output has changed to a very structured and demanding system of progressive workouts and her estimated caloric output is between 2,500-3,000 calories each day.

Yet she refuses to move from an 800-calorie diet because of fear. Her active output demanded more energy, but her caloric and nutrition intake was insufficient. How will the body make up this deficit? It will affect the internal structures and convert energy there. Muscle mass is converted, glycogen stores are depleted, and the sympathetic nervous system is activated and likely the cause for a compromised immune system.

I lost track of how often I have worked with someone stuck in this trap. They get their workouts dialed and execute flawlessly each week only to not see results. Their fear is causing this and if they just trust the obvious, they nearly always see improvement in a matter of days. But getting a young woman off the 800 calories to a more reasonable 2,000 is a coaching challenge.

Effectively, I am asking these ladies to nearly double their habitual intake, and this takes time to overcome. I can say that in my experience over the years, every woman that slowly increased her intake of nutrient-dense foods saw fantastic results because their fitness was already dialed. Once the nutrition comes into play, the results come as well. But it is very scary for these people who have imposed this rigid idea that fewer calories equal better results. They don't.

Fear of Guilt

By my observation, the fear of guilt seems to manifest in two specific forms. On the one hand, some feel guilty before they even start and saturate their thoughts with self-doubt, questioning their decisions and feeling generally dissatisfied. On the other hand, I have seen some people allow guilt to drive an obsessive-like adherence to certain aspects of a program.

This is especially true with extreme calorie and food journaling. In both cases, guilt drives a strong feeling of responsibility for the outcome, and shame gets tied into the feelings of guilt even if there is not a perceivable failure. As a foundational principle, I suggest caloric counting and exercise adherence be a well-constructed, yet flexible guide based on discipline, not an obsession.

Having stated that, I commonly see the first group where doubt and indecisiveness cause paralysis, and that results in feeling guilty, because of the indecisiveness and lack of execution. The guilt is usually because the person feels like they are on the wrong path, or their problems are so big that they can't seem to solve them no matter how hard they try. Guilt comes in the form of missing workouts or slipping up on food.

It is common for someone to overeat at lunch and then just throw the rest of the day away and binge because they felt they already failed. Guilt is especially strong where someone is suffering from an eating disorder and can't seem to defeat it. The feelings of being so completely controlled by something like anorexia, bulimia, obsessive macro, and calorie counting, or other disorders often cause many people to get stuck in the cycle.

Look at bulimia, for example. Guilt fuels a binge, guilt fuels a purge, guilt fuels self-loathing, then guilt triggers binging, and it repeats. I have worked with dozens of women and men stuck in a cycle, and they are hesitant to start any program because they fear if they pay attention to it, they will obsess on it and the cycle will activate. Sadly, many of their needs exceed my scope of practice, so I refer them to a clinician, but I still support the basics of a designed exercise plan for these clients in conjunction with a mental health caregiver if they choose to do so.

It's heartbreaking how many stories I could share around this topic, and if you experience these feelings or are suffering from an eating disorder, know there is hope, and you can get out of the cycle. It is hard, and you may have relapses and feelings of defeat, but I have seen so many people pull themselves out of this destructive situation. You can do it, so never give up.

One of my favorite clients suffers aggressively from bulimia with intense feelings of guilt, fear, and shame. She has struggled from the time she was a teenager and is now in her early 30s but still fighting. Some of our coaching calls are just letting her cry and work through her thoughts. She has several awesome weeks, and suddenly, she will message me letting me know she spent the last two days binging and purging to the point of exhaustion.

I must modify her workouts often to accommodate and help support her needs as best I can. Her clinician has had her stop food journaling for reasons related to obsessive-compulsive disorder, and we reduced her workouts to low impact just to keep the habit of working out. Plus, she always feels better after exercise, and we have found that strength training is one of her new favorites, and she is less likely to skip.

She particularly loves circuit training because we can do it in a half-hour and she need not think, she can just do it. She is working on overcoming this intense guilt and finding her internal strength.

A special note to her: You light the lives of others, and your value is immeasurable. Your quality is not dictated by the past and the pain there, it is in the future you are making. Find your joy.

Fear of Exhaustion

And here we come to my personal fear-based habit resistance, and I suspect it is shared by millions of hard-working people. For me, it's not so much about the habit of exercise, but more about knowing I have been working twelve or more hours and still need to complete my workout. I must be very sharp for my client calls, writing, research, and programming and it is easy to resist the structure of planned workouts and justify based on time and exhaustion.

I already tend towards insomnia, so that compounds the fear of feeling drained. I see this in almost all my clients to some degree and there are several strategies to overcome this fear. Remember that we can tie excuses such as not having enough time to this as well, but in the end, it's about avoiding the feeling of depletion.

This is a simple fear to overcome, but it is not easy. Time management, prioritization, and shifting one's mind to make wellness an inclusive part of their life can be quite challenging in practice. However, I have never met anyone who can truly justify a lack of time as a reason to not work out.

There are 168 hours in a week, and you most certainly can find thirty minutes to an hour every other day in there. Let's say you committed to five, 30-minute workouts each week, you still have 165.5 hours left. Even if you slept for only six hours each night, you still have 123.5 hours. Of course, you are an extremely hard worker and put in long hours professionally with an average workaday of twelve hours over six of the seven days in the week, leaving 51.5 hours.

You are very committed to friends and family, so each day you spend at least five hours with loved ones ringing in 35 hours. This leaves you 16.5 hours weekly, which is 2 extra hours each day.

So why is it you can't seem to fit in exercise? Well, it's not about time, it's about exhaustion or lack of prioritization. Occasionally the fear of exhaustion is tied to laziness and lack of willingness.

Chapter Keynotes

The primary intention of this chapter is to help readers understand the basics of how a habit is formed. Moreover, this chapter helps you identify and understand the various forms of resistance that can interfere with your efforts to change. Resistance comes in several flavors, but they all end in self-sabotage and delayed results.

- Habits are an acquired set of behaviors that have become almost involuntary, rooted deep in our subconscious through patterns and instigated responses.
- Generalized habits alone are not good or bad, but the nature of the habit can be classified one way, or another based on your relationship with the activity.
- Habits create continuity, efficiencies, and reward in our daily activities.
- Diverting energies to affecting personal change based on your projected outcome will be critical for success.
- With positive wellness-based habit formation, we must apply a deliberate set of actions based on a known instigator, a planned response, and a reward in line with our outcome objective.
- Even though we all know change is inevitable, we resist because it pulls us out of homeostasis, removes predictability, and instigates the fear of loss.
- Oscillation is essentially a massive overcorrection, which leads to negative feedback and regression.
- We must be careful not to apply selective knowledge to our habit alteration journey as this is a self-limiting practice.
- Do not become emotionally connected to specific approaches and resist change even if what may have been effective for a period, is now producing little or no return.
- The comfort of predictability and pain we already know can sabotage the development of healthy habits if we perceive change as painful or uncomfortable.

- Fear-born anxiety is double-edged because it can inspire action or cause paralysis, so it is important to courageously meet fears head-on and address the source of your resistance and act.
- We must eliminate the fear of disruption by addressing solutions that will resolve the negative consequences of our behavior.
- Be aware of procrastination as it reinforces our fear, and we justify why we can't seem to make our fitness and nutrition efforts payoff.
- To avoid feelings of guilt, I suggest caloric counting and exercise adherence be a well-constructed, yet flexible guide based on discipline, not an obsession.
- Time management can be instrumental in avoiding or limiting feelings of exhaustion, which stifles habit change.

"

AUTHORS PERSONAL NOTE

At some point, it occurred to me that I did not have a fitness or nutrition problem. I had an attitude problem. Once I fixed that, everything else aligned.

Chapter Three
THE 30X3+10 RULE

In fitness and nutrition circles, we often hear about what percentage of our results come from exercise versus what comes from diet. The most popular seems to be the 80/20 split, whereas 80% of your expected results come from your nutrition and only 20% from your activity. Another take on the 80/20 split is that 80% of our food should be healthy and nutritious, but you can certainly indulge in 20% less than healthy foods and be fine.

Beating this drum again, I suspect people gravitate towards diets because exercising is hard and takes time, and you can try a new diet pretty much overnight. In my experience, people seem more likely to alter their diet and happily ignore activity.

This makes the 80/20 split looks attractive and easy to slip into. I have even heard some coaches, nutritionists, social media influencers and people subscribed to a dogmatic diet, claim exercise is not even necessary. But let's examine that claim: "With a proper diet, you can get results, so exercise is useless."

The fallacious claim that exercise is useless without nutrition is a weak argument because it begs the question and makes several assumptions. The premise is that exercise is useless but evades the debate by emphasizing "with a proper diet, you can get results." This conveniently glosses over the controversial part of the argument that exercise is useless, which is being assumed.

This also perfectly sets up a false dichotomy for people pushing pills, diet fads, and gimmicks. They are saying there are only two choices, and we might as well buy the easy approach of diet or a pill because we can get results with just a fad or supplements so ditch the workouts. And once again, they use this as a marketing strategy in an appeal to low effort on behalf of the consumer.

Anyhow, these arguments have little merit and do not serve most people. Proof can be found in hundreds of studies conducted related to the obesity epidemic in the United States. Look at the Center for Disease Control and Prevention website if you need to confirm, we are getting fatter.

In the argument above, we also assume exercise is simply for weight loss or aesthetics, yet neither should be a primary motivator to work out anyway. The premise overlooks intrinsic benefits of exercise such as the reduced risk of disease, cognitive function, mood enhancement, energy balance, sleep, libido, strength, mobility, endurance, connective tissue health, bone density, circulatory health, and so on.

This means I don't buy into this 80/20 thing, and I most certainly do not advocate a sedentary lifestyle. So, what percent comes from fitness and nutrition? Well, I don't think it comes down to one or the other. I believe it is about combining and acknowledging four specific aspects: Attitude, Nutrition, Fitness, and Genetics, which make up what I call the 30x3+10 Rule. Remember, this is a sliding scale, but all these components represent a unique percentage for everyone.

For example, a small fraction of people can maintain an excellent attitude about their fitness and nutrition but may lack knowledge or structure. Some people can manage their nutrition well but struggle with exercise or keep a negative attitude about it.

Conversely, some people can nail their workouts but just can't seem to get the food part down. Slide these percentages to your own needs but know that the 10% genetics cannot move. You have very little control regarding genetics, so attitude becomes even more important when addressing aspects of your life in which you have little power.

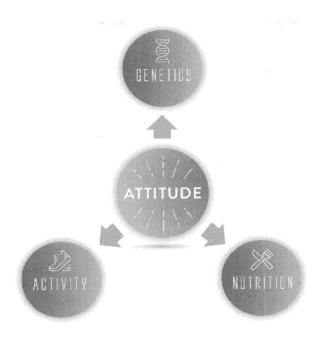

Attitude = 30%

"We want a Ferrari for a body, but some treat theirs like a salvaged 1987 Buick Sentry and then complain when it breaks down."

We can call this mindset or attitude, and it typically represents 30% of your overall wellness and should be addressed before you even start a diet or exercise program. You can have a perfect workout plan that is world-class or a clinically constructed meal plan and still fail. You must get your attitude about wellness focused into a proactive thoughtfulness about where you are and where you want to go.

You must plan and organize your life, so wellness becomes inclusive and not some abstract inconvenience that comes around every January for a short time. I would say that nine out of ten clients that start with me have an attitude problem, not a fitness or nutrition problem. Occasionally, I get a new client with a positive attitude that just needs some help refining their workouts or food lifestyle, but that is rare.

I must spend time in each of the first few coaching sessions with new clients exploring mindset so I can understand motivators, goals, and the desired level to make their objectives a reality. We must break the cycle of fitness failure, and the first place to start is in how we view wellness and the way it impacts our lives. In our modern world, we are mostly stuck in high-stress jobs, sedentary personal lives padded with historically unprecedented levels of comfort.

Our food sources are calorie-rich, nutrient-poor, suspiciously manufactured, and are alarmingly convenient. We do not have the luxury of disconnecting ourselves from managing our activity or our food choices if we want to control our wellness. I often hear people claim they don't have time, energy, or desire to exercise or eat appropriately. What they usually mean is that they have not made wellness a priority and hold it at arm's length but are unhappy and have a bad attitude about it.

I like to ask new clients, "What have you tried in the past, and has anything been successful for you?" The typical answer is, "Yes, of course, I have tried the XYZ diet and lost twenty pounds." My response is then, "And have you maintained that loss?" And nearly every single time, the answer is, "No, I even gained it all back plus an extra ten, so I am up thirty pounds." I use this as an example to show the incredible resistance we demonstrate toward sustainable lifestyles and taking personal responsibility for our wellbeing.

Instead, we "try" a fad diet or gimmick but end up miserable all the while. It also shows we never address the root cause, which this book is intended to help you correct. We just generally get a sour attitude about it all, and that compounds resistance. For years we neglect ourselves, carelessly consume low nutrition foods, and remain inactive but then want the sea to part and heavens to rain down huge fat loss because we just bought a new diet program we will abandon in a month. It's ridiculous.

"This is the one," you tell yourself, "This time I am going to stick with it because that multi-level marketing nutritionist on the YouTube said if I buy their super juice smoothie and just cut out all red meat, grains, lectins, gluten and hang upside down eating kumquats I can lose twenty pounds in one month." Sold!

We must make wellness inclusive to our whole life and not hold it out at a distance. The reality is we must align our attitude and recognize that the things we blame for obstructing us from being able to manage our fitness or food, such as our career or relationships, will directly suffer from a lack of wellness.

Your professional and personal life suffers when you are unwell. Your performance, health, vitality, patience and focus all diminish. Your capacity to be the spouse, parent, friend, manager, employee, entrepreneur, or student you want to be is compromised by a lack of wellness. We must prioritize our fitness so we can perform to our maximum capacity in these things.

We must take care of ourselves, so we may take care of others. But this means you must get your mindset aligned to self-care and learn to take great joy in exercise and feeding your body with wholesome foods. Self-love is the gateway to an improved attitude about wellness and acknowledging the reality that fitness and food management are now a necessity in our sedentary world of high convenience and low nutrition food sources.

If you love and take care of yourself, then workouts become exciting, and eating well and nutritiously brings even more joy. Self-love also includes how we speak to ourselves inside our minds. Negative or destructive internal comments and putdowns accumulate, and you will believe your pessimistic assertions. I touch on internal self-talk in several other places within this book as it is a critical component to developing a strong internal attitude.

I will give two examples illustrating the difference between mindset and attitude. First, let's look at how mindset can affect your outcome. For over a year now, I have worked with a highly intelligent and driven woman who struggles to include her wellness in her high-stress life. Her mindset was divided because she placed her personal and professional life in silos and off in the distance, she quarantined her self-care.

She works as a high-level manager and is pursuing an additional graduate degree to advance her career. She is married and works to balance her relationship and family. In her intense focus on her career and keeping her personal relationships, she neglected her body. Inevitably, her body abandoned her as well, and she was stuck in a cycle of acute injury and became overweight.

She tried several times over the years to get back on track and reduce her body fat and improve her musculature to ease the tension in her joints and the pain in her body. As a military veteran and driven professional, she would try extremes such as going from sedentary to suddenly running a marathon. Unfortunately, this just wore her down even more and she became stuck in an injury cycle.

Yet her mindset was not inclusive, and her attempts were not rooted in sustainability. She just went extreme with the hope it would jolt her back into a better fitness lifestyle and food relationship. The constant injury and feelings of exhaustion caused extra stress with studies, work, and even her relationships for a time. She could not see how her wellbeing was the key to her personal and professional success.

Her mindset was that she needed to focus on school, career, and spouse before she could think about herself. I also learned over our sessions she had some deep feelings of not being good enough or she was a failure. On the contrary, this woman is anything but. Yet, her mindset would not allow her to see her total value and her level of self-love was quite low. She did not prioritize her wellness because she felt she did not deserve it and was responsible for taking care of others first.

She has been working very hard to bring fitness and nutrition back into her daily awareness and make it part of her so she can be strong, energetic, and sound enough to perform and be the best she can in her life. On our coaching calls, she mentions how she feels so much better after a workout and how her chronic pain is not as sharp.

When I wrote this, she has not had a relapse into injury for several months. She is still trying to reign in nutrition but is doing better all the time. She is working to break down the walls between herself and the silo she built around her wellbeing. She is shifting her mindset towards making her fitness part of her and not just something she does when she has time. She is making time.

The second scenario is all about a positive attitude. I have hundreds, perhaps thousands of stories about clients with negative attitudes and pre-conceived failure. But I want to share an uplifting story about how keeping a positive attitude can make all the difference. I work with a gentleman who is a small business owner, husband, and father.

He is extremely busy, but his mindset is that to perform at his best, he needed to get fit. He was already working out regularly but was just not seeing any return on the time spent. He tried all sorts of programs and was very dedicated, but his body was not responding to the template workouts he found online. This was his motivator to contact me so we could custom build a program and make adaptations as he progressed.

From day one, this guy was on fire and ready to jump in. He had already decided that he would give 100% to the workouts and get his food on track and be joyful about it. Despite the fact for the last year, he was working out with little to show in results, he checked his attitude. We started with some basic metabolic conditioning and foundational lifts to get him ready for more work and changed his program every four weeks based on his biofeedback and measurements.

He never complained about workouts but would ask great questions if he was unsure why we were doing something, but after I gave him a brief scientific overview to renationalize, he just attacked the workouts without complaint. He is proof that home gyms can work because he gets up every morning, checks in, and crushes every single day. He has set boundaries with his family and expressed how important this is for his vitality and goes into the garage and gets to work, mostly uninterrupted.

He has profoundly transformed his performance and physique in the last seven months, and just today, as I write his story, he told me it is translating professionally. His energy when meeting with the staff has become contagious, and he feels his positive approach and feeling of confidence have set a new tone for his company culture. His shirts fit tight, his shoulders are back, head high and he is full of joy for his life and how he feels each day.

In all the time we have been working together, he has had only a few small moments where he needed some encouragement. Recently, he has had several compliments about his bearing, and he sent me a message recently saying, "I have had multiple people comment on my physique lately. One guy even told me you look swole. That feels really good, but what they don't see is the seven months of busting my ass."

Like I said in an earlier chapter, you can buy into a program, but if you do not do the work, you can bet your results will be zero. Yes, it is hard work, but nothing is greater than improving oneself. When you have a strong mindset and positive attitude, you can overcome any obstacle and the outcome will be worth it every single time. If you have a reclusive mindset or a negative attitude, there is not a diet plan or workout type out there that will do you any good long term.

Nutrition = 30%

"Nearly all the mainstream fad diet plans share an identical formula which is highly restrictive caloric recommendations, elimination or reduction of a macronutrient and the over glorification of a single or set of food sources. It is a trap."

Proper nutrition is simply the sum of food source quality, nutrient density, and total caloric value evaluated each day tied into a proactive awareness. There is no question, nutrition management is fundamentally key to sustainable wellness. It is true, you cannot outwork poor food choices, but this does not mean nutrition is more important than exercise. Remember, we established that without the right mindset, the likelihood of long-term success is greatly diminished in both diets and workouts.

We see this disconnection of mindset time and again with fad and crash diet program failures and regressions. How many diets have you tried? In my experience, I have found that a calorically appropriate and well-balanced food lifestyle is the most successful and sustainable.

Everyone has their preferences and food reaction combination. The trick is to find the optimal food lifestyle for yourself. I like to start by creating a baseline by identifying the likely energy output of a client, then construct a meal plan that delivers the energy needs of their activity and daily life.

I start with a simple ratio of around 40% carbohydrates, 30% protein, and 30% fats and adjust based on biofeedback and lifestyle. I estimate calorie suggestions on their cumulative fitness goals because nutritional requirements will be quite different for a twenty-four-year-old male competitive bodybuilder over that of a sixty-five-year-old woman with a hip replacement. Take the time to educate yourself from reputable sources and be aware of how your body responds to foods.

In Part Three of this book, I break down the basics of nutrition and outline dozens of strategies for nutrition success. You must take responsibility for learning the fundamentals of how carbohydrates, proteins, and fats affect the body along with understating basic energy balance.

You don't need a fancy diet plan or some system of restriction, you need to educate and experiment with your responses to food type and volume. Do not obsess over calories and the ratio of nutrition as that will not serve you sustainably and healthily unless you are in the top 1% of performance athletes.

Instead, I encourage you to see food as a gift of energy and a means to provide your body and mind with the fuel to succeed. Yes, you must be aware of your intake and not exceed your daily need, but occasionally one can have planned indulgences. This is completely reasonable, provided you maintain a level of conscious consumption and limit the volume or duration of the excess. If you have a plan and it fits your intended outcome, then you are in a position of power and can manage the occasional treat. If you are not yet there, then stay the course and work on your Wellness Consciousness.

One of the biggest obstacles many of us must overcome is our unhealthy relationship with food and diet concepts. We have explored the falsehood and negative aspects of fad diets in the previous chapter, so let's look at food relationships first because this is often tied to an internal or external instigator. One of my very long-time clients works as an influential and successful executive with a dizzying schedule.

Over the years, we have worked to get her aligned with a strong mindset and joyful attitude about exercise and a better relationship with trigger foods despite her travel and stress. She mostly has mindset, fitness, and acknowledgment of genetics under control, but nutrition had a set of challenges. In her office, long morning meetings are a regular occurrence.

For some time, she struggled with the presence of doughnuts in these meetings. Her habit was to unconsciously take a doughnut at the beginning of each meeting and depending on the length, she may occasionally indulge in two doughnuts. She pointed this out during a coaching session as one of her external instigators and the morning doughnut was something she wanted to limit or remove from her habit. In her situation, she did not want to effect change by eliminating doughnuts in meetings even though she had the authority to make that happen.

Instead, we overrode her internal habit, so she had a higher level of Conscious Response and could control the external presence of the doughnut temptation. We began with altering the habit by employing a timing and weaning strategy. This is extremely helpful by creating awareness and deliberate acknowledgment of the instigator while reducing the withdrawal or feeling of deprivation. We started the habit alteration with two specific approaches.

First, she would wait until the meeting was approximately half over before she made a move to get a doughnut. Second, if she did get a doughnut, she would cut it and only take half. The idea was to move the instigation from the start of a meeting to break the mindless habit of walking in and grabbing a doughnut. She must now walk in, acknowledge the instigator, and deliberately not engage the old habit.

By reducing the serving size, she was altering the habit of consuming a full doughnut so she could get her sugar craving under control with less risk of relapse. Over time, she reduced the serving to a quarter, and eventually, she was able to ignore the doughnuts completely and now only partakes when she decides to indulge. This is a perfect example of a topic we will cover in a later chapter called Wellness Consciousness.

To give you a sneak peek into this concept, she started in a state of Careless Unconsciousness, where she was not thinking about her action. Suddenly, she made a Conscious Realization and wanted to make a change more attuned to her intended outcome. Doughnuts were not part of that. She then moved her mindset into Conscious Action, which was the deployment of a defined strategy to reduce and hopefully eliminate the draw of the doughnuts. She overcame an environmental instigator and now must work at consciously maintaining it.

Today, she feels much better and more "in control" when there are food instigators present because she has made this awareness part of her normal habit when in meetings or even at parties. Food holds a significant set of instigators for most people, so we must be very conscientious about these risks. They can be triggered by emotional events, stress, environments, peer pressure, nostalgia, or just mindless consumption.

Nutrition management is not just about calories, macros, and food type, it is also about your mindset and awareness related to it. When you combine a positive attitude and mindfulness with a calorically appropriate and nutritious food lifestyle, you already have 60% of the work done. Now we need to tie in your activity.

Activity = 30%

"When we think about working out, we tend to imagine grueling exercise. Yet exercise is simply the structure that allows us to predict an outcome. Activity is the total expression of energy and relates to the sum of proactive wellness. Be active and be well."

Activity is not just exercise; it is the total value of your daily expenditure. This includes the level of effort required in your career, at home, and in your recreational preferences. Exercise is wonderful because we can apply a specific set of stressors to the body and get a predictable outcome. If you want to be a sprinter, then you train like a sprinter, not a marathon runner.

This is because we can predict physiological adaptations based on structured stress. Sprinters work on fast-twitch muscle fibers, phosphagen, and glycolytic systems along with speed and power training.

Marathon runners work to improve slow-twitch muscle activations, oxidative stress tolerance, lactate threshold, and cardiovascular endurance. One of the biggest mistakes people make in their structured exercise is applying the incorrect stressors for their desired goals.

You can read more about building appropriate workouts and learn to avoid that pitfall in Part Three of this book. Anyway, the point is activity and exercise are not the same things in an abstract way.

Exercise is critical if you have specific performance or aesthetic goals, but total activity is a component of your daily energy output. The more active you are, the more effectively your body utilizes nutrition and the more neuromuscular benefits you will enjoy.

Humans are made to move, and our bodies do not thrive in low-activity environments or sitting all day. This is apparent in the obesity epidemic and the growing problem with movement pattern dysfunction from poor posture. I advocate for structured exercise based on your condition and goals coupled with an active lifestyle. This means you have a formal workout plan for specific results, and you make additional decisions to activate your body.

This includes parking further from the door at work, taking the stairs, adding a brisk daily walk, getting involved in a sport or training for a 5k, and so on. Personally, I am an avid backcountry hiker in all seasons save winter. Training for these hikes does not necessarily replace my workouts, they supplement my total activity. Hiking is just my chosen active recreation and I seamlessly integrate it into my regular workouts. Rock climbing is also part of my active lifestyle and does not replace structured exercise.

I do, however, move workouts around to accommodate added activity now and again. If I have a long hike coming up on a weekend, I swap leg day from Friday to Wednesday. If I am rock climbing, I will move my back or biceps exercises to not interfere, so I am fresh for the walls. In spring, summer, and fall, I add supplemental walks that can be over five miles.

On these walks, I always listen to an audiobook. This way I can activate my body and mind in the same hour. As a benefit, I typically get through around sixty or so books each year. I also listen at double speed, so that helps. I see activity as a whole picture and not fragments of time spent in a gym, and if you prioritize wellbeing, this is quite simple and enjoyable.

Genetics = 10%

"We all have a genetic potential. The first trick is deciding how close you want to get to that potential, the second is finding satisfaction when you get there and the third is maintaining it."

Genetics include height, gender, body type, potential, and predisposition for disease or other biological realities outside of your direct control. For this book, we will focus on the physiological structures and not dig so much into the medical consequences of genetics.

One of the major issues I have seen emerge over the years is when someone has a genetic disposition in opposition to their specific goal. This means they do not possess the specific Somatotype as the person they are inspired to emulate.

Somatotypes are a classification theory for the genetic disposition of physiological structure and include ectomorphic, mesomorphic, and endomorphic frames. Somatotypes were developed in the 1940s by Dr. William Sheldon, a psychologist trying to link body type to personality.

His assertion that physiological structure can be a predictor for behavior has been disputed and in my opinion, absurd, but his classification of body type remains popular today. I am only pointing out his physiological classification and the Heath-Carter Formula used to calculate anthropometrical measurements to determine body type, not personality.

An ectomorph is typically tall and thin with a narrow body, long arms, and legs, little or low body fat, and long muscles. An example of an ectomorphic person would be a basketball player, long-distance runner, or fashion model.

A typical mesomorph would have a sturdy build with a broad muscular chest and shoulders, naturally muscular arms and legs, and little natural body fat. An example of a mesomorphic person would be a gymnast, bodybuilder, or physique competitor.

An endomorph is generally thick or stocky, with a large round body, thick arms and legs, and a tendency to store body fat if not diligent. Examples of an endomorphic person are a football lineman, powerlifters, or every guy cast as a bouncer in a movie, except Patrick Swayze in Roadhouse. Like most notable male dancers, he was a strong blend of mesomorphic with some dominant ectomorphic traits.

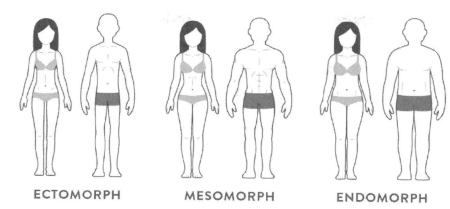

ECTOMORPH   MESOMORPH   ENDOMORPH

There are degrees of divergence within each body type, so be objective about your primary disposition and find ways to be the best you can despite the uncontrollable.

Based on the Heath-Carter equation, there is some opportunity for an ectomorphic person who works hard and trains specifically to improve physique may move slightly closer to a mesomorphic appearance. Conversely, an endomorphic person can train to reduce body fat while optimizing performance and appearance with the right training application.

However, there are limitations and levels of maintenance required to move from a baseline body type towards some features of another. You cannot change your genetic body type, but you most certainly can enhance it to be the best it can be, and that may loosely resemble one type or another.

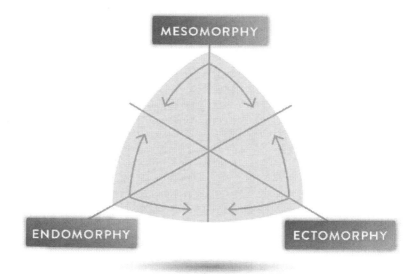

As I mentioned, many people have a vision for their appearance at odds with their genetic disposition. I see this all the time in male and female clients, and it can be a difficult conversation to have. To be clear, while you may have a genetic disposition you do not find favorable, you can move your aesthetics to some degree with the right workouts and food intake.

No, a heavily ectomorphic man standing at five-foot-nine will never have the physique of a strongly mesomorphic man standing at six-foot-three. Nor will an endomorphic woman who stands at five-foot-two look like an ectomorphic runway model standing over six feet. To drive this point home, you may not control your baseline body type, but you control your attitude about it and how well you have constructed your fitness and nutrition to be the best version of yourself.

I will share my personal story of frustration, disappointment, and acceptance of my body. In 2012, I was going through some serious life changes, and at the time, I was running my consulting firm in the morning and teaching advanced fitness and nutrition sciences for Bryan University in the afternoon. This left me with several hours during the day, and I used the time to work towards my maximal genetic potential.

I was excited to hone my body to its highest level of conditioning and aesthetics, so I wrote out a highly specialized training plan and dialed in my nutrition expertly. In my head, I envisioned my five-foot-ten frame holding layers of rippling muscle and single-digit body fat percentages. My workouts consisted of over an hour of resistance training five to six days each week with progressive loading and heavy hypertrophy work.

I would also take another hour at least six days a week for some light cardio such as long walks, bringing total structured exercise time over two hours each day. Rest and sleep patterns were planned and specific to ensure adequate recovery. Nutrition was hyper-focused, and all foods were well-sourced, calorically appropriate, and nutritionally dense. I ceased all alcohol consumption, eliminated added sugar completely, and consumed over two pounds of vegetables daily.

My protein intake was from whole food sources only, so I was not using supplements to reach or exceed 0.08 grams per pound of bodyweight daily. Fats were mostly mono and polyunsaturated with carbohydrates that were low glycemic, and undulating based on training intensity. I was relentless and diligent. After the first year, I found that while I was finally in single-digit body fat percentages, my lean tissue was lagging. I was about 158 lbs at 9% body fat and stuck at about 140 lbs of muscle.

I was very lean and muscle striations and vascularity were impressive, but I was quite small. Ok, not to worry, I just needed to adjust my program, so I reworked my fitness approach and added more calories and protein to my intake. For nearly six months, I worked as hard as I could to get over 160 lbs, but instead, I dropped to 150 lbs and 5-6% body fat. Wrong direction. I stopped all intense cardio and focused exclusively on heavy lifting and added in some powerlifting techniques to inspire some mass adaptations.

Six months go by, and I get from 150 lbs back to about 159 lbs keeping at 6% body fat or less. I was the only guy I knew at the time that was sub 160 lbs that would rep 4 sets of 6 deadlifts at

380 lbs with excellent form. I was two years into the most intense training program and specialized food intake only to realize that no matter how hard I worked, my ectomorphic body would not evolve into a mesomorphic one. Damn.

I was seriously frustrated. I worked harder than anyone I knew, and the results were not what I expected. I then had some of my colleagues at the University look at my micro, macro, and mezzo training formula to get secondary professional advice. Nope, it all looked good except for one small problem. I was trying to get a heavy mesomorphic outcome without the genetic capacity for it. I got bitter and the frustration drove me to try and lift even heavier.

As a consequence of my inability to accept that my body looked remarkably fit, and my strength was inhuman for my size, I went even harder. My reward was a class-one biceps tendon tear in both arms when curling 120 lbs on a bent bar.

My initial discipline had turned into an obsession, and I paid the price with an injury that still affects me today. I now have clicking and discomfort every time I do any bicep work and developed chronic lateral epicondylitis. These self-inflicted injuries have fundamentally changed how and what I can lift.

I had essentially reached my genetic potential and once I got there, I was dissatisfied and disappointed. This experience has helped me reconcile my capacity, and I have since learned to love my body and fully embrace what I can do with it, not what I cannot. When I look at photos from that time, I am overwhelmed with the realization I suffered from dysmorphia and was so obviously fit to the point of exceptional. Why the hell did I not see or appreciate it then?

Because I had an unrealistic expectation and was unwilling to allow that my genetic potential was not what I envisioned. Instead of feeling a deep sense of accomplishment for molding my body into its potential, I was resentful.

I will never allow this negativity to poison me again and now fully embrace my body and understand my genetics are not within my control, but I can maximize the gifts I have.

I will never be over 200 lbs of muscle but have found that with a more tempered and sustainable approach, I can move my body to some semblance of mesomorphic. This is particularly true in my chest and triceps, but that is about it. And I am profoundly grateful that I have found joy and peace with my body and work to make it all it can be.

Now, I acknowledge that there is a small percentage of people whose genetic makeup interferes with their fitness results or wellness. However, using genetics as an excuse for ignoring your activity and negligent consumption is unreasonable and a weak justification for poor choices. I have observed a substantial increase in using genetics as an excuse over the past few years, and it's just another copout.

Yes, genetic factors may present certain challenges or change how you approach your wellness, but that means it may be even more important to get your activity and nutrition dialed in. If a genetic disposition elevates your risk of disease or decreases performance, then you must mitigate that by focusing on your wellness and not use it as an excuse for mismanaging your health.

Chapter Keynotes

The body will follow the mind so if you have a poor attitude or layers of resistance, you may be self-inflicting needless suffering. This includes your attitude regarding managing your fitness levels and food relationships. Finding joy in our unique genetic disposition and potential while discovering ways to maximize that potential is empowering. We all tend to be critical of our bodies, but I encourage you to reconcile what you can control as opposed to what you cannot.

- Attitude, Nutrition, Fitness, and Genetics, which make up what I call the 30x3+10 Rule.
- This is a sliding scale because all these components represent a unique percentage for everyone.
- You must get your attitude about wellness-focused into proactive thoughtfulness about where you are and where you want to go.
- The reality is we must align our attitude and recognize that the things we blame for obstructing us from being able to manage our fitness or food, such as our career or relationships, will directly suffer from a lack of wellness.
- Negative or destructive internal comments and putdowns accumulate, and you will believe your negative assertions.
- It is true, you cannot outwork poor food choices, but this does not mean nutrition is more important than exercise.
- Take the time to educate yourself from reputable sources and be aware of how your body responds to foods.
- I encourage you to see food as a gift of energy and a means to provide your body and mind with the fuel to succeed.
- Exercise is wonderful because we can apply a specific set of stressors to the body and get a predictable outcome.
- The more active you are, the more effectively your body utilizes nutrition and the more neuromuscular benefits you will enjoy.

- I advocate for structured exercise based on your condition and goals coupled with an active lifestyle.
- Somatotypes are a classification for the genetic disposition of physiological structure and include ectomorphic, mesomorphic, and endomorphic frames.
- There are degrees of divergence within each body type, so be objective about your primary disposition and find ways to be the best you can despite the uncontrollable.
- You cannot change your genetic body type, but you most certainly can enhance it to be the best it can be, and that may loosely resemble one type or another.
- Using genetics as an excuse for ignoring your activity and negligent consumption is unreasonable and a weak justification for poor choices.
- In the end, your success in fitness and nutrition will come down to your attitude about your body and your willingness to correct destructive habits.

AUTHORS PERSONAL NOTE

I understand change is inevitable and the growth potential of my life. I will embrace change and master my responses and avoid hiding behind fear, doubt, or obstinance. Today, I decide to embrace change.

Chapter Four
STAGES OF CHANGE

Now that we have discussed some of the conditions in the media and the fitness industry, habit basics, and limiting beliefs, let us talk about the Stages of Change. We will uncover negative internal and external instigators and develop a solution for each in the 90-Day Habit Workbook, but first, you must know where you are in your mindset and attitude towards wellness.

This is so you can formulate a specific strategy to get where you want to go. For any individual to maintain fitness, they must have already decided to be successful and keep an objective attitude about the process. In a more technical sense, we look to the Transtheoretical Model of Behavior Change (Prochaska & DiClemente, 1984, 1986, 1992). Traditionally, behavior change is often construed as an event, such as quitting smoking, drinking, or overeating.

However, we should recognize change as a process that unfolds over time, involving progress through a series of stages. While progression through the Stages of Change can occur linearly, a nonlinear progression is most common. Let's take a brief look at each of these stages and spend a few moments to reflect and identify where you fall into this cycle. In Part Two of this book, you will work to identify your position in the Stages of Change along with space for you to outline the specific habits so you can create a strategy for change.

My experience has led me to identify complexities in the stages of change and I understand how hard it is to layer subtle changes that manifest into real sustainability. I encourage you to consider where you stand in the stage of change as it relates to your fitness & nutrition mindset and willingness to improve. I suggest you take notes as you read Part One of this book to assist your thought process while filling out any of the workbook portions in Part Two.

This is so you may grasp some of the major points and become more granular with your thoughts after absorbing some of the key concepts of behavior change and conscious response. I just want to expose you to some of the hard questions you must ask yourself, so it's in the back of your mind as you read and see where you land in the Stages of Change.

Precontemplation

Individuals in the Precontemplation stage do not intend to act in the foreseeable future, usually measured as the next six months. In general, people who are underinformed about the consequences of behavior or just ignoring them are found in the Precontemplation stage. In addition, these people have typically gathered multiple unsuccessful attempts at change, which can lead to demoralization about the ability to change.

It is highly unlikely any person in the Precontemplation stage is even reading this book, and if you are, you likely are one of the folks that have been unsuccessful with change in the past. Also, you may know people in your life at this stage. I point this out because it can make a difference if your support system, such as a spouse, cannot see your perspective and need for change.

Contemplation

Contemplation is the stage in which people intend to change in the next six months or so. These people are usually more aware of the benefits of changing but are also acutely aware of and dwell on the disadvantages. This is where it can be frustrating because, in fitness, people are comparing an unhealthy lifestyle against a healthier lifestyle. Making this comparison is a nonsensical thought process.

There are no advantages to an unhealthy lifestyle when compared to a healthy one. Some would argue the advantage of an unhealthy lifestyle is that you get to eat whatever you want. This is a farce as eating what you wanted is what got you in this problem to start with and your declining health or excess fat is a consequence, not an advantage. Plus, many people in this situation have had repeated failures with long-lasting fitness or nutrition behavior change.

It is quite interesting because people will make a conscious decision not to change in favor of living fit and instead choose poor nutrition or a less active life and remain miserable and discontented. Comparing the benefit and costs of changing can create ambivalence, so people will stay in this stage for extended periods.

This phenomenon is often characterized as chronic contemplation or behavioral procrastination and there is a correlation with the obesity epidemic. Yet this is the stage where contemplation for change happens, and awareness is evident. If you feel this is a stage you are in, there are several things you can do to emotionally engage and inspire preparation.

Preparation

Preparation is the stage in which people intend to act in the immediate future and they may have already taken some steps toward positive change in the past year. These individuals have a plan of action, such as joining a gym, hiring a coach or personal trainer, or diligently working on a self-managed approach.

These people are ready to take significant action. However, buying into a program differs from executing it. I tell folks all the time, you can buy 100% into a program financially, but if you do only 1% of the work, you will fail. People in this phase will sometimes try and buy fitness.

Expensive trainers, programs, gyms, or equipment for their home makes them feel like they started. Usually, there is little follow-up or action taken and inevitably, they quit before they started. You cannot buy fitness. It is an action and life discipline, not a new car.

Action

Action is the stage in which people have made serious or significant positive modifications to their lifestyles. However, to qualify as true action, individuals must be in the stage for at least six months, or they were really in the Preparation phase the whole time. Because action can be observed and quantified, the overall process of behavior change is often associated with an action.

However, the foundations of action started long before the execution of an idea or goal takes place, and most people who start an exercise program do not make it six months. In the fitness reality, these stages of change can be a bit cyclical because once we achieve our primary objective, we must work to maintain it, and therefore, there are elevated chances of lapse or relapse. It is my goal to help you make it past six months and create a sustainable fitness lifestyle.

Maintenance

Maintenance is the stage in which people have successfully altered behavior, the action has produced results and they are working to prevent relapse. While in the Maintenance stage, people are less tempted to relapse and grow increasingly more confident they can sustain their new behavior and habits.

In addition, many people see a new manifestation of goals from an elevated or improved lifestyle, such as new athletic endeavors, outdoor activities, or another life-enhancing enterprise. You should continue to monitor behavior in some objective fashion. Journaling is a great way to keep a record and compare trends related to instigators.

Environmental management and keeping a clean house will go a long way to support you. Most importantly, keeping a conscious and deliberate set of responses to your known triggers while looking at every instigator as an opportunity. I welcome instigators because it allows me to practice my behavior or habit alteration and maintain resolution in acquisition and response.

Chapter Keynotes

Humans love to daydream about their future, success, and lifestyle. This comes in a vast range of needs because we are all different and do not universally share the same life situation. But we all daydream about having it better.

Sadly, when it comes to wellness, most people seem unwilling to change even when they identify their pain points, and the solution is within reach. Some have tried to make that personal change but for whatever reason, they failed and have become discouraged.

- For any individual to maintain fitness, they must have already decided to be successful and keep an objective attitude about the process.
- There are no advantages to an unhealthy lifestyle when compared to a healthy one.
- We should recognize change as a process that unfolds over time, involving progress through a series of stages.
- I encourage you to consider where you stand in the stage of change as it relates to your fitness & nutrition mindset and willingness to improve.
- Individuals in the Precontemplation stage do not intend to act in the foreseeable future, usually measured as the next six months.
- Contemplation is the stage in which people intend to change in the next six months or so.
- Preparation is the stage in which people intend to act in the immediate future and they may have already taken some steps toward positive change in the past year.
- Action is the stage in which people have made serious or significant positive modifications to their lifestyles.
- Maintenance is the stage in which people have successfully altered behavior, the action has produced results and they are working to prevent relapse.

" "

AUTHORS PERSONAL NOTE

Empowerment is not something we can reliably obtain from an external source or person. True empowerment is taking control of our behavior and internal dialogue. Self-Empowerment inevitably leads to higher levels of consciousness and personal mastery.

Chapter Five
WELLNESS CONSCIOUSNESS

I have created a basic model for understanding where we are in our level of personal awareness and the ability to alter learned responses. I call this concept the "4 Stages of Wellness Consciousness." In clinical psychology, there is a model for consciousness and level of competence. This is similar as it relates to a level of awareness in stages, but this is less abstract and more of a guide with actionable steps.

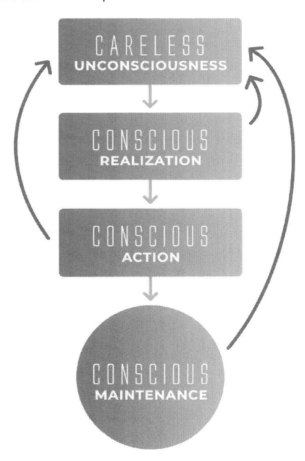

Stage One: Careless Unconsciousness

This is the common stage for individuals disconnected from their habit patterns and instigated behaviors. We carelessly wander through life, relying on a set of destructive subconscious reactions we have learned to help us cope or automate. Usually, this carelessness can be related to a strong emotional impulse, desire for instant gratification, or self-protection mechanism.

It is hard to identify when we are in this stage because the problems and habits are so much a part of our reactionary responses. We find ourselves in various periods of dissatisfaction and often, we can even pinpoint a condition resulting from our Careless Unconsciousness but lack the facility to solve the problem to some degree.

For example, stepping on a scale and getting a disappointing result is the byproduct of Careless Unconsciousness and not the root cause. However, we identify the emotional pain from the scale and ignore what behaviors got us there. We just focus on the weight number and superficially make a weak resolution to improve our diets or start working out, but rarely is this acted upon or sustained.

Evidence is in the obesity and overfat populations along with the growing number of deconditioned individuals. Unfortunately, the stage of Careless Unconsciousness can last long periods, and often, becomes permanent, causing us to get completely paralyzed within it.

Stage Two: Conscious Realization

In this stage, we have suddenly realized that we are not in the desired state physically or emotionally as it relates to our wellness. Jeans don't fit, mirrors tell painful truths, and we just feel awful. We have realized and made a conscious connection, and this sets us up to act. This stage is powerful as there are only two outcomes. Either we revert to Careless Unconsciousness, or we move on to the next phase of Conscious Action.

In this section, let's examine the trap of reverting to Careless Unconsciousness where many of us get stuck and repeat that cycle over great periods. An example is joining a gym or going on the next big diet only to quit within weeks or months. This is troubling because so many people agonize in this cycle. We make a realization and take some type of action to recover our constructive actions only to fail. This reinforces fitness failure and creates a festering sense of hopelessness. We fall back into our carelessness and disconnect from our daily awareness and sink deeper into our suffering.

Of course, we will repeat the cycle through our lives if we allow it and always carry the burden of dissatisfaction with all the demons that accompany it. The second outcome is the ability to make the conscious realization and create within ourselves the mental fortitude to persevere to the Constructive Action phase. Success comes from more than realizing and deciding to act. Success comes from identifying and addressing habits that led to dissatisfaction in the first place.

You can have the greatest fitness plan in the world developed by a Master Personal Trainer, or a nutrition plan guided by a Registered Dietitian and still fail. This is because programs only work when you do! But hard work is a fast-burning fuel, and there must be more substance to your mindset other than just beating yourself up at the gym or making better food choices. For long-term success, we must address the hard stuff and connect our minds and bodies so we can sustain action and alter habits.

One of the temporary consequences surrounding a newly elevated consciousness and realization is how it illuminates aspects of our behavior that can be embarrassing or cause a feeling of remorse. Unfavorable behavior discoveries are part of the process and should be embraced to overcome the negative action. It is important not to reinforce a negative self-perception as this relates directly to the principle of positive internal conversations.

Past behaviors are where you were, not where you are going so, cast off the embarrassment or remorse and solve the problem through Conscious Action.

I find on some nights I struggle to sleep; my mind wanders back to historical personal or professional events, and I replay mistakes I have made in my lifetime. This is only constructive if you use these memories as a reminder to avoid the same mistakes in the future. It does not serve to ruminate on your past, so be mindful that your Conscious Realizations are used to fuel personal improvement, not get stuck in feelings of regret.

Stage Three: Conscious Action

This stage ties into the planned response notion we will review in the next chapter called "The Power of Conscious Response" but it is worth preemptively expanding upon here. We react instinctually in many areas of our lives, and I propose we take a moment and plan a response in the areas we wish to improve.

Naturally, positive behaviors or normal daily activities can be autonomous. I am suggesting we deliberate on our choice of action or words when instigated by a discernible emotional instigator. I have worked extremely hard over the years seeking to improve my planned responses based on conditions or environments that antagonize me.

Like all worthwhile pursuits, Conscious Action takes practice and consistency. I have observed the more that we practice these principles, the easier it is to create a proactively positive internal headspace and, to some degree, influence our external environment to accommodate goals.

Remember, Conscious Action should be well constructed and thoughtful. Aggressive overcorrections are not always a conscious action, they are conscious reactions, and like overcorrecting in a vehicle, the results can be disastrous.

Some of your action items may be quick and simple fixes, while others may take a fair amount of time and steps to correct. This is where managing your expectations and understanding the dynamics at play make the journey more rewarding and reasonable, so be patient with the complexity of self-improvement.

Stage Four: Conscious Maintenance

Life circumstances are always in flux, so conditions or instigators can also change suddenly. We must vigilantly manage our perceptions to skillfully maintain agility in our response. In our modern world of high stimulus and the opportunity for dynamic life changes, we can never disengage from the principles of conscious thought.

If we detach from a deliberate response in our targeted areas of self-improvement, we place ourselves at risk for relapse into old habits or create new undesirable behaviors and revert to Careless Unconsciousness once again. Like exercise, the powers of conscious response must be maintained, or the results degrade.

Wellness Action and Consequence

In our pursuit of self-improvement, we must combine the Power of Conscious Response and continually identify our stage of Wellness Consciousness. However, acknowledgment and awareness are void without action. Because sustainability is one of the primary intentions of this book, we must examine constructive and destructive action duration.

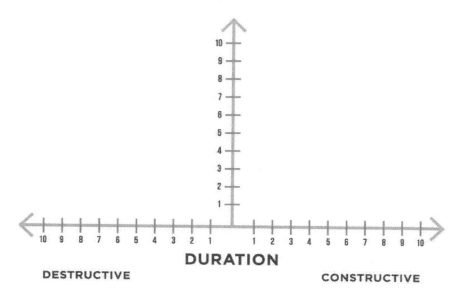

Constructive Action

Constructive action is when we plan, execute, maintain, and review our behaviors to compare against our goals or intended outcome. Constructive actions start with a positive mindset that easily translates to exercise adherence and proper management of nutrition. Planning is critical because if there is a small lapse, you have a guideline for getting back on track.

Destructive Action

Destructive action is when we get off track, neglect exercise, over-indulge, experience self-doubt, or feel guilty, and so on. This starts when we neglect or abandon our plan, but we can certainly be in the destructive action phase with or without a plan. Many people are perpetually taking destructive action. Without a plan, they have no waypoints to guide them, so the duration can extend into despair.

Behavior Intensity (Y)

The level of intensity must be considered for both constructive and destructive actions. On the Y-axis, we can estimate the total impact our choices or automated behaviors have on our intended outcome. We then compare to the X-axis, which is Behavior Duration. It is the combination of these two factors that determine the total value of constructive or destructive action.

Behavior Duration (X)

The success of constructive action can be measured by the time you can maintain the duration of these positive behaviors on an X-axis. Likewise, the damage from destructive action is the combination of intensity and duration towards negative outcomes. We should strive to make this a lifelong success and not revert to a destructive state, but that may not be realistic. Thus, the key is to limit the duration in which you may slip into destructive action.

Behavior Planning

Now that you understand how the damage caused by a lapse can be determined by the time and intensity of destructive actions, we must develop intended outcomes to validate progress.

If you currently have a decisive plan and you fall from the constructive action phase, suck it up buttercup, and get back on the trail quickly. You have a map, so you know the way. If you do not have a plan, then make one and be aware of when destructive actions take place and limit intensity and duration.

The most common and simple example I see of a minor yet potentially devastating destructive action comes from when someone eats in excess at one meal and says, "Well, I already screwed up so I might as well keep going and eat whatever."

The intensity and duration of this mindset plus the resulting behaviors determine the total damage. Common sense argues one should say, "Well. I screwed up on this meal, so I must be extra vigilant the rest of the day."

But no, that is not the "common" response to a minor lapse as many people will spend a good deal of time in a destructive state. The goal here is to elevate your wellness consciousness and avoid or reduce time in destruction. This becomes particularly powerful when you have developed specific intended outcomes.

I encourage you to objectively look at these components of your life at least once weekly. I have made it a practice to take a Saturday or Sunday morning and compare my constructive and destructive actions over the past week to my intended outcome and seek ways to improve deliberately.

This is extraordinarily helpful when making weekly attitude adjustments and can help you overcome feelings of guilt, disappointment, or resenting the process. Let us look at an example tied to food. Say for the last week, you were dialed in on your nutrition with whole foods, low sugar intake, and appropriate calorie consumption. You can evaluate the intensity or Y-axis and draw out for seven days to create a box within the level of intensity and duration.

Now let us say you have been invited to a party over the weekend and you indulge and overconsume. You must stop and acknowledge the intensity and duration before you submit to negative mindset automation. In our example, you already have one whole week of positive constructive food management. Now we need to determine the level of intensity and duration of the overindulgence at the party.

In our example, we can use the Y-axis of intensity plus duration on the X-axis and square it. You can even draw this on a graph and shade in the sum of the intensity duration line into a box. Do the same for the past week of constructive food action. If you were to superimpose the shaded portion of the destructive behavior over the week of constructive action, you will see the total impact of the destructive compared to constructive behaviors.

In this case, you will notice the destructive action is a mere fraction of the sum of constructive action. So why would we focus and dwell negatively on the small and often insignificant destructive action? You have a whole week of incredible constructive behavior so let go of the minor overindulgence and all the negative thoughts around it. It's comparably insignificant to the constructive aspect of your week as illustrated below.

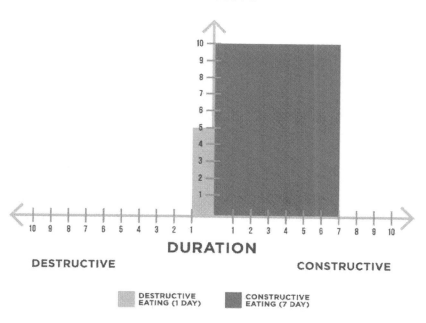

Chapter Keynotes

The 4 Stages of Wellness Consciousness serve as a model for understanding where we are in our level of personal awareness and improves our ability to alter learned responses. Wellness Action and Consequence is the awareness and objective measurement of Destructive versus Constructive action. Combining an elevated wellness consciousness and the ability to assess destructive or constructive action give you the tools to plan behavior and overwrite undesirable habits.

- Careless Unconsciousness is the common stage for individuals disconnected from their habit patterns and instigated behaviors.
- Usually, this carelessness can be related to a strong emotional impulse, desire for instant gratification, or self-protection mechanism.
- It is hard to identify when we are in this stage because the problems and habits are deeply ingrained into our reactionary responses.
- In Conscious Realization, we identify that we are not in the desired state physically or emotionally as it relates to our wellness or life vision.
- Conscious Realization is powerful as there are only two outcomes. Either we revert to Careless Unconsciousness, or we move on to the next phase of Conscious Action.
- Don't get stuck in feelings of remorse as your conscious realizations manifest. Past behaviors are where you were, not where you are going so, cast off the embarrassment or remorse and solve the problem through Conscious Action.
- Conscious Action is kinetic, deliberate, and requires planned responses to known instigators exposed by Conscious Realization.
- Naturally, positive behaviors or normal daily activities can be autonomous. I am suggesting we deliberate on our

choice of action or words when instigated by a discernible emotional instigator.

- Conscious Action should be well constructed and thoughtful. Aggressive overcorrections are not always a conscious action, they are a conscious reaction.
- Some of your action items may be quick and simple fixes, while others may take a fair amount of time and steps to correct but all habit improvements will require maintenance.
- We must vigilantly manage our perceptions to skillfully maintain agility in our response.
- If we detach from a deliberate response in our targeted areas of self-improvement, we place ourselves at risk for relapse into old habits or create new undesirable behaviors and revert to Careless Unconsciousness once again.
- Because sustainability is one of the primary intentions of this book, we must examine constructive and destructive action duration.
- Constructive action is when we plan, execute, maintain, and review our behaviors to compare against our goals or intended outcome.
- Destructive action is when we get off track, neglect exercise, over-indulge, experience self-doubt, or feel guilty, and so on.
- The level of intensity must be considered for both constructive and destructive actions.
- The behavior duration of constructive or destructive actions should be viewed objectively.
- I suggest daily and weekly comparisons of the intensity and duration of both constructive and destructive actions.
- The goal is to have more constructive actions than destructive but when there is destructive behavior, you must resolve to overcome and move on.

AUTHORS PERSONAL NOTE

"

I control my thoughts, feelings, and actions. I am the master of my mind and own my body. I am aware, thoughtful, and deliberate in my actions. I will not allow external forces to control me. I will not allow my negative thoughts to control me. I will be kind, gracious, and loving to others and most importantly, to myself.

Chapter Six
THE POWER OF CONSCIOUS RESPONSE

Now that we have a better understanding of the Stages of Change, let's look at the mechanics of what it takes to create a real, sustainable fitness and nutrition lifestyle by improving our mindset and altering habits. I learned the concept of conscious response the hard way in 2006.

The forthcoming personal and slightly embarrassing story demonstrates a direct correlation between making a meaningful discovery in one area of our life that can be applied to other aspects. In this story, a career situation started the process of personal improvement that translated to a universal focus on my conscious response, behavior choices, and mindful habit alteration.

I had just left my managerial role at a major international chain of gyms and became the Vice President of a struggling high-end country-club-style fitness company in California. The two companies had quite different models and therefore, attracted certain kinds of employee demographics.

Over the previous five years, I had developed a set of learned responses and a leadership approach commensurate to the culture of the well-known international chain gym. The widely accepted management style of this organization was extremely aggressive and hyper-focused on sales and productivity.

I was hired by the high-end fitness company specifically to correct the revenue issues and improve operational quality, especially with member acquisition and personal trainers. I was young and excited to be part of a company course correction, but this reasonable exuberance was deemed too aggressive by many in the new organization.

Sadly, the staff of the new company had already passed judgment on me before my first day. When the news was released that I was joining the team, many employees and managers formally complained about my past five years as they believed I would bring the industry-renowned intensity from my former employer. The bias was already there, and I could feel it from day one.

While I certainly did temper my learned response style as a professional, it was not enough to overcome the culture. Every disciplinary action I had to take against an employee for any reason reinforced the bias of the staff, managers, and my fellow executives, which further alienated me.

Any operational changes or improvements were met with resistance and suspicion. To be clear, the company was already struggling financially, and much of this was because of the overwhelming amount of destructive nepotism, entitlement, broken departmental operations, and poor-performing employees.

I identified that I must adapt my responses and be far more conscious about word choice and tone to effect change in my new environment. As I said, it was not enough and perhaps too late to improve the perception others had formed of me early on, but I decided to frame this concept of conscious response and apply it more deliberately. The interesting and unexpected result of taking time to think about responses or decisions was the translation to other aspects of my life.

Unfortunately, while I was slowly concluding conscious response, my deep feeling of frustration by how the staff unjustifiably perceived me and the undermining actions of peers provoked my unconscious self to make destructive choices.

This was greatly compounded by significant challenges developing in my marriage. At this point, I was now dealing with a crushing amount of both professional and personal turmoil. To cope, I would pour an ounce of scotch or a glass of wine at the end of, particularly hard workdays. But the habit reinforced as time and repetition went on and then it grew from one cocktail to several on these tough days.

The habit manifested further and grew to several days each week. Over time, it exploded into a glass of scotch or wine every single weekday after work, and I doubled down on weekends. Scary, it was the first thing I did when I got home. In a twist of irony, I suddenly realized over nearly two years of a high-stress life situation I had become lazy with my workouts and had been making poor food choices as well.

I was not only drinking too much alcohol, but I had also become overweight by my standard. There I was, a certified personal trainer and fitness company executive and well over 25% body fat with bad habits. When the heck did this happen? How did I not catch this or act to correct this earlier? The simple reality is once I unlocked my conscious and deliberate behavior, my error was exposed.

Plus, I could hide my growing waistline in a suit and began to even dress to conceal my situation. Even so, I knew my trousers were getting very snug, I was skipping workouts, and the recycle bin was mostly wine bottles, but I had relegated it to my unconscious daily justifications. I was too busy, tired, and whatever other excuses we all conjure to rationalize behavior.

I understood then I had to act and make highly focused and specific personal goals and set some boundaries for myself. That is when I started to outline the process to do just that so I could visualize and apply actions to get back on track and form some better habits. This is when I developed The Power of Conscious Response model for myself.

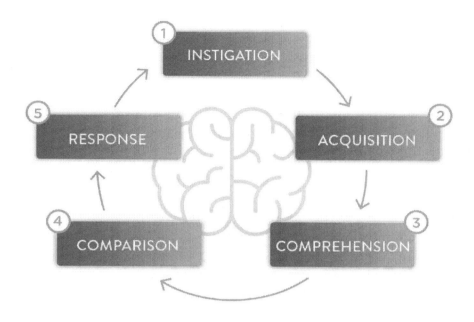

Conscious mastery over one's tendencies or habitual response is an essential concept regarding the Power of Conscious Response. This also requires awareness about one's emotional reactions to instigation.

Those with intense emotional responses without comprehension can typically cause unnecessary personal tension or engage in behaviors that reinforce bad habits. The acquisition phase is so important because it is the gatekeeper between instigator and comprehension.

For most responses, we neglect comprehension and comparison, so our reactions are unplanned, and dominant-negative habits prevail as a response. Here is how the cycle of Instigation, Acquisition, Comprehension, Comparison, and Response applied to my story:

Behavior Instigation

Action instigators can be internal thoughts and feelings or external stimulation that provoke a response. Instigators include words, tone, implications, sights, scents, sounds, or any stimulus that instigates an unconscious and automated reaction. Instigators and habitual reactions can be classified as positive or negative depending on their effect on your life, so take time to identify your unique instigators so you may formulate planned and optimized responses.

Be warned, sometimes we do not recognize the instigator straight away or proactively deal with it as it is received. We often hold on to it, and the energy from that instigation is released later in private or once the situation has passed. This release is nearly always in the form of a destructive or undesirable coping habit such as excessive alcohol consumption or binge eating.

Instigation in Action

In my confession earlier, the instigation was when I would overhear or have it reported to me the unjust, dishonest, and hurtful things staff or peers were whispering to each other about me and the direction of the company.

At the time, I felt deeply wounded that my effort to improve reputation and perception was unilaterally disallowed. Even the CEO of the company would incite conflict between me and other executives, managers, or staff when he wanted to preserve a relationship with one of them.

He would use me to discipline and terminate employees so other managers and he could save face because "they were all friends." This was enormously stressful for me and quite uncomfortable. It would also undermine any goodwill I managed to accumulate with staff, and I felt completely suppressed. This caused me to look for reward behaviors, and it turned out to be a cocktail after a long day.

Funny thing is, I was about twenty-five years old when I had my first cocktail, and I was never a big drinker. Go figure. The cautionary tale here is that bad habits can manifest from unlikely places, and even though alcohol was never previously part of my life, it silently crept in.

Instigator Acquisition

We receive and subconsciously process information from internal sources and external sensory information daily. In most of these unconscious instances, we have yet to comprehend the instigator, and our core personality traits or automated habits often manifest and provide a response. This would be what I think of as a habitual response without conscious consideration.

Acquisition in Action

In my story, I share the escalation of my evening cocktail habit. Notice it took reinforced and unconscious actions to accumulate into a full destructive force. I was painfully unaware and just simply looking for a reward or compensation for my situation like most people do with food, sex, risky behavior, alcohol, or worse. It is the reward component that makes a habit so damn strong and tough to identify and break.

I had not yet even comprehended that I had formed a destructive habit as the pleasure of instant gratification overrode any ability to make the connection. This is where Acquisition is the gatekeeper between the stimulus and comprehension of actions. I was able to transition out of the Acquisition phase into the Comprehension phase because I had decided to increase the resolution of my conscious thinking in a seemingly unrelated aspect of my life. In my story, the trigger and the remedy turned out to be the same thing in the end.

I was making bad habit choices because I felt hopeless in my career, yet in my attempt to improve that career, I became aware of the bad habits developing in my life out of coincidence. Of course, this is likely very uncommon, and your triggers or instigators may have little or no connection to how you concluded elevating conscious thought and response.

What matters is the identification and acknowledgment of a habit you wish to overwrite and then apply your attention to change. Fundamentally, you need to comprehend you are doing it.

Instigator Comprehension

An instigated sensory cue is often benign to our consciousness until it is comprehended. Mostly, we just move to the habitual response and skip comprehension and comparison. Comprehension is the point of deliberate internal decision-making for action or to combat a rote habit.

This is the challenging aspect of elevating your consciousness to accept and process information or sensation because it requires thought and deliberation. Taking a moment to acknowledge and comprehend that you have been given a sensory cue is the foundation for developing responses in line with your target personality and outcome.

This is where we write new responses and over time, they can become a habit we purposefully install and overwrite the former undesirable habit. Applying awareness and equal parts patience are necessary to navigate comprehension.

Comprehension in Action

I comprehended the unintended consequences of poor choices and the resulting habit formation after I slowed down the process of internal and external trigger response. When I truly took a moment to analyze an instigator, I sorted the risk factor and let the insignificant stuff go. This allowed me to focus more intensely on the cue that would activate my subconscious response of pouring a cocktail or glass of wine.

I was able to quickly identify specific types of triggers and then resolve to overcome my learned behavior. Plus, by rejecting the insignificant or trivial triggers, I found a great deal of peace. It was difficult initially as the habit was rooted, and I could expect a relatively instant reward from the drink habit compared to the temporary low-yield reward of disciplined behavior management.

Like a memory, habits never really disappear, so we must remain vigilant and keep our consciousness sharp. They will always loom in the background, ready to emerge and reinsert themselves if we are not careful. Comprehension is the key to real, lasting change along with the acknowledgment, but not acceptance, of forces that drive an objectionable action. If you accept your condition, then you have not elevated your thoughtfulness to the degree where you will change.

I had to decide, with strong conviction, to reduce my consumption and find alternative positive reward outcomes to replace the negative habit. To gain this conviction, you must make a comparison to your vision of self, and we do this in the Comparison phase.

However, after this initial revelation and successful overwriting of weekday drinking, I have had to course correct one other time in recent years. Stay vigilant, and do not let the old habits reemerge. If they do, just repeat the steps, and affirm to yourself that you did it once, you will recover again.

Habit Comparison

We need to make a comparison before we integrate intentional action by comparing the response to our internal desires and beliefs. This is when emotional, moral, or principal comparisons are made against a comprehended instigation. This includes comprehension of pending undesirable physical and emotional damage. Compare an instigator to your desired outcome and intentionally develop responses that meet your behavior objective.

Simply, you must be true to who you want to be, and when your moral compass is aligned with your planned responses, you will believe in them and fortify your resolve. It is awfully hard to create habits or behaviors if they are antagonistic to your belief or bias structure. Yet, we can exert remarkable control over our personalities even if the progress is slow and takes time. People can change if they take conscious action to make that change.

Comparison in Action

In my example story, I had realized that being over fat, making poor food choices and weekday drinking was outside of my life plan. I had to compare the rewards and consequences of these behaviors to my set of personal evolving morals and principles. Did I want to be an out-of-shape fitness professional?

Did I want to feed my body with low-quality foods? Did I want to move from a bad habit of weekday drinking to alcoholism? Did I want to allow others to instigate me to this degree?

It was so clear once I made the conscious realization the answer to all these questions was an unequivocal "No."

Ask yourself similar questions about habits or behaviors you wish to correct. Take firm action against your negative or self-destructive habits by developing positive responses.

Conscious Response

Behavioral responses are formulated once an antagonistic force is received, comprehended, and compared to instinct, knowledge, and bias. Subconscious reactions become evident here because they are the product of habit and practiced response. A response can be any reaction that is perceivable such as action behaviors, expression, tone, or language used to reply to an instigator.

Action behaviors are kinetic and relate to a more physical response, such as binging on ice cream after receiving an instigator. The idea is to replace the negative behavior of consuming ice cream as a response with positive behavior, such as working out or listening to an uplifting song. As a side note: expression, tone, and word choice are more of a third-party perceivable behavior and usually occur in relationships or professional environments.

Response in Action

Now that I had completely exposed my foolishness and poor choices for coping, I was challenged to find a planned response. I realized the factors in my professional and personal life were adding tremendous stress, and the habitual response was to seek a stiff drink or make a poor food choice to avoid pain and supplement pleasure.

Ok, so now what? I had to make a concerted mental drive to acknowledge when I was at risk and then have a prepared response. In my case, I turned to audiobooks and a sixty-minute powerwalk.

When I got home, I would ignore the liquor cabinet or refrigerator and immediately change into workout clothes. I had a book downloaded and ready to go. I would step outside and make a mental confirmation I was choosing this as a reward over my previous habit. I was willfully overriding past behavior and affirming that action consciously.

Here are several rewards I enjoyed from active and conscious responses. First, I reduced my overall alcohol intake dramatically and only imbibed during the weekends in a controlled fashion. Second, I lost fat at a significant rate. In the first six months, I went from 219 lbs to 175 lbs with an average fat loss of 1.5-2.0 lbs weekly. I got that down to 155 lbs and 8% body fat within a year and a few months. Third, I was reading or listening to over five books per month, so I was enhancing my education. Fourth, I found more productive ways to consciously manage my responses at work, and this improved conditions in my career to some degree.

Finally, this experience gave me a new empathy for folks struggling with habit alteration, body fat loss, or personal development. It made me a more effective personal trainer and coach because I was able to specifically outline the process for change and appreciated the challenges many of my clients face. I believe my suffering made me a better coach and leader, so now I optimistically embrace challenges.

The pain of this experience and my ability to overcome negative behaviors have translated into many aspects of my life and while I have encountered new points of pain, I have the formula to overcome them.

Of course, my responses are not perfect, and I am still on the path to higher conscious thought and planned response. Yet, I feel far more equipped and empowered to manage a reply to my internal conversations and the things outside my control. I have also found now that I have taken greater control of how I react, I feel less anxiety, feelings of failure, or discontentment. You can too.

Positive Events May Be Instigators

I used a personal example of a life situation that was undesirable to illustrate the concept, but instigators are not always negative at their source. Jovial aspects of life can also be powerful instigators and emotional catalysts. The Holiday season is a great example of a positive instigator for most people and the results turn negative.

The New England Journal of Medicine estimates that the average American gains several pounds of fat between Thanksgiving and New Year's alone. This is where the Power of Conscious Response becomes a tool to maximize your positive life experiences without diluting them with negative outcomes. By creating a personal awareness and strategy to navigate, you can effectively enhance the exciting aspects of life without attaching unintended consequences.

Therefore, we must elevate our mindfulness, and we can do that through the 4 Stages of Wellness Consciousness outlined in the previous chapter.

Chapter Keynotes

Actively engaging in your internal and external instigator response is a critical step towards slowing or stopping destructive automated habits.

- Behavior Instigation, Instigator Acquisition, Instigator Comprehension, Habit Comparison make up the cycle of Conscious Response.
- Mastery over one's tendencies or habitual automation is an essential concept regarding the Power of Conscious Response and requires awareness about one's emotional reactions to Instigation.
- The Acquisition phase is important because it is the gatekeeper between instigators and Comprehension.
- For most responses, we neglect Comprehension and Comparison, so our reactions are unplanned, and dominant-negative habits prevail as a Response.
- Action instigators can be internal thoughts and feelings or external stimulation that provoke a response.
- Instigators and habitual reactions can be classified as positive or negative depending on their effect on your life, so taking time to identify your unique instigators so you may formulate planned and optimized responses.
- We receive and subconsciously process information from internal sources and external sensory information daily.
- In most of these unconscious instances, we have yet to comprehend the instigator, and our core personality traits or automated habits often manifest and provide a response.
- An instigated sensory cue is often benign to our consciousness until it is comprehended.
- Comprehension is the point of deliberate internal decision-making for action or to combat a rote habit.

- Taking a moment to acknowledge and comprehend that you have been given a sensory cue is the foundation for developing responses in line with your target personality and outcome.
- We need to make a comparison before we integrate intentional action by comparing the response to our internal desires and beliefs.
- You must be true to who you want to be, and when your moral compass is aligned with your planned responses, you will believe in them and fortify your resolve.
- Behavioral responses are formulated once an antagonistic force is received, comprehended, and compared to instinct, knowledge, and bias.
- Action behaviors are kinetic and relate to a more physical response, such as binging on ice cream after receiving an instigator.
- The idea is to replace the negative behavior of consuming ice cream as a response with a positive behavior.
- By creating a personal awareness and strategy to navigate, you can effectively enhance the exciting aspects of life without attaching unintended consequences.

"

We so often get stuck in the routine of our existence that we rarely stop to truly develop a plan for our growth and fix on a destination. We merely wander through life or go with the flow and hope it takes us somewhere we can be happy. It never will unless you take control and drive towards your intended outcome.

Chapter Seven
DEVELOPING INTENDED OUTCOMES

In my own life, I have worked to envision my optimal physical self and personality. I have developed a projected intended outcome for my life I am working towards every day. My intended outcome is self-actualizing and a prime intrinsic motivator and allows me to stay on target, mostly.

This chapter is the product of watching thousands of people over the years taking their potential influence and personality for granted or simply ignoring their self-improvement. Bear with me on this topic as I want to explore the dynamics of influence and how this can support your ability to manage external environments more effectively.

We must prioritize our personal development to affect our automated behavior, habit imprints, and improve conscious response. I feel it important we cover some concepts intended to improve your perception of yourself and thus, improve the perception of others.

To some degree, the perception of others is fundamental to improving your external environment and because we do not live in a closed system, we must be aware of how we affect people in our circle. Through the power of attraction, you can greatly influence others and the support system they may provide. This ties back to instigator management.

Having acknowledged the dynamics of perception, I believe the growing popularity of the copout phrase "perception is reality" or any similar sentence exposes an ignorant or narcissistic attitude.

I have noticed the accelerating trend of people justifying their incomplete thoughts, feelings, failures, mistakes or just making excuses or pardoning themselves from constructive dialogue or actions by using this kind of phrase. It's annoying to observe and will damage your potential.

When people cling to their own bias and perceptions, they are displaying an entitled and limited perspective, which is self-hindering and eliminates potential proactive debate, resolution, and personal growth.

If you subscribe to that kind of egocentric mindset, you are saying: "Hey, all that matters are me and my perspectives so, my special perception is reality and your views, thoughts or feelings do not matter."

It's a weak and arrogant way to justify exclusion and ignore personal responsibility and is corrosive to constructive social and professional relationships. If you expect to be a person of reasonable influence and success who can develop their life outcomes, you must be willing to examine multiple perspectives and compare to your bias and see if there is room for you to modify and progress your mindset, which is a shift in perspective.

If you do this with a positive attitude, you have created a new reality, so don't get attached to linear thinking. Perception changes with information, time, environment, and experience. Therefore, perception is temporary for those seeking self-improvement. Sustainable habit alteration requires we be willing to change perspective so we can be objective about our behavior and assess potential destructive actions and correct them.

To sum it up, here is an example: You and a friend are out for a walk, and you look up and see the sky is a beautiful vivid blue. Your friend, who suffers from a form of color blindness looks up and says, "Wow, look at how clear this green sky is today!" For the sake of the example, let's assume around 8% or less of the world is color blind and sees blue as green, but the vast majority sees blue. What perception is reality?

You and your friend continue to walk, and you produce a pair of special color correcting lenses that turn greens to blue. You have your friend with the green perspective look through them. Now what? With a new environment, the green turns blue, so perception changed but has this changed reality? Well, 8% is not a strong case for the inflexibility of perception when 92% see blue. Do not get attached to your perceptions or you will always be blinded, and it will be hard to F.I.N.D your way.

The F.I.N.D Principle

F - Focus your Passion
I - Invest in your Personality
N - Navigate with Agility
D - Develop Perseverance

Let us look at four components that drive your intended outcomes and set the stage for successfully improving your sphere of influence or external environment. I call this the F.I.N.D. Principle. The power of a dynamic personality is simply that of attraction.

When you focus on improving these areas, a natural byproduct is often an enhanced sense of self-love. I like to simplify the character traits that form an attractive personality by narrowing down the popular adjectives and attributes to those that hold the greatest endearing power.

Any opportunity to emerge as a positive force within your sphere of influence is predicated upon whether you possess a strong magnetism. To peel away the layers and complexity of this subject, I am speaking about influential dynamic energies and engaging communication. A positive influencer works to win the hearts and minds of those around them and can communicate and connect with a broad spectrum of personalities.

Consider a previous chapter where we explored internal and external instigators and life modalities related to behavior. We get instigated and must mindfully choose how to respond to that trigger. My point is, when you have true passion, you become intrinsically motivated and likely to succeed because the purpose of your actions transcends the end reward. The behavior backed by a personal passion is its very own reward and can shape your evolving personality to some degree.

If we maintain agility in our direction and avoid obstinance, we can course-correct quickly and stay on track. Determination or perseverance is often a byproduct of activities rooted in a personal passion and drives you through difficult periods of discomfort or hardship, making success more likely. By proactively and consciously creating a strong personality, you can affect the two environments that produce opportunities for good or bad decisions.

First, our internal environments, in which we leverage the greatest control. Second, our external environments, in which we do not possess the same degree of control. However, by developing a lifestyle and set of attractive and powerful personality traits, we can greatly influence both environments and therefore mitigate many instigation opportunities. When we love ourselves, we trust ourselves and the risk for relapse is reduced.

Conversely, when we love others and reinforce this with positive behaviors, love is often reciprocated thus creating a strong system of support. Hopefully, we have generated an internal and external support mechanism and platform for improvement in both environments. The good news is we all have the power over our internal environments and can make incredible improvements to ourselves.

How do you "find" your way? What happens when your external environment will not respond to your influences? Do you change your environment? Do you change your attitude towards it? Or do you simply ignore the negative aspects of the external and focus on the controllable? When you have a strong personal baseline, you can answer that question for yourself.

Focus your Passion

I define passion as an intense, convicting force that drives the desire to participate and, in this case, the passion to develop lasting fitness and nutrition habits. To be widely effective, the term passion must be focused and inclusive to each component of what shapes a successful set of behaviors.

This means one must possess a sincere passion for the definitive values and traits that form the basis of their wellness success. It also means we must focus our passions, so the potency of it resonates into results. A prime factor in this formula is self-actualization and the desire to make personal improvements.

These traits, founded on passionate self-love include preparation, action, and setting goals that are focused and attainable. Successful personal improvement objectives must have specific and measurable goals for the reinforcement of positive habits through results or rewards.

Be warned, casting a wide net may not always be an effective use of passion as it can dilute effort. We must prioritize our efforts to maximize the usage of passion energies.

In the same manner, a personal trainer designs an exercise program for clients, a prudently constructed habit change program should be marked with starting points, milestones, acknowledgments, and opportunities for adaptation. By developing a concise plan and means to check your progress objectively, you can improve and validate progress.

Action is the kinetic component of change and evidence of true self-love. Action is also the catalyst of visible results fueled by our foundational passion for self-improvement because an emotion or goal is useless without action. We must liberate ourselves and passionately pursue our objectives. Plans or personal goals collecting dust and devoid of focused behaviors delivering action will prove nothing more than wasted dreams and lost ideas.

To expound that point, passion or energy withheld and restricted to the heart and mind of the individual is benign to the universe and will simply dissipate and absorb into the subconscious of the holder as action opportunity appears and then passes. All those hopes and dreams will simply corrode, dull, and fade with the merciless advance of time. Fear, doubt, and laziness act as a barrier between the raging swells of positive emotional energy in your mind and the action potential of your being.

This limiting barrier must be broken down, so your passion is unfettered and free to drive your potential toward your focused and intended outcome. When action is applied with a passion to a plan, then a result will likely occur. But it is those who are wise and aware that will recognize the degree or direction of results and compare it to an objective and make adaptations accordingly.

Therefore, we must remember not all results are necessarily aligned with our careful planning or congenial to intention. Do not become overly discouraged by the unpredictable nature of results. Stay the course of success yet learn to circumnavigate and not become mired in the jagged rocks of disappointment. To maximize effectiveness, preparation and action require you to become passionate about personal improvement.

It would serve poorly to abandon or suspend a well-designed personal plan by behaving inconsistently with a lack of passion or action. Inconsistent behavior also muddles momentum, stifles energy, and may erode your internal personal trust. Consistency coupled with results will generate self-trust, but not following through with your plans will erode that self-trust.

You must believe yourself when you say you will do something and the only way to ensure this is to do it. If you set yourself up to fail, then inevitably, your behaviors will not result in your intended outcome. Your plans must not be so broad that your budding passion for healing is inadequate fuel between milestones. The world is unpredictable, and action produces results and consequences that may not be foreseen or avoidable.

We must prepare to have our plan challenged by life events and have contingencies to remain vigilant and retain self-trust. I would argue the risk is worth the reward when passion, action, and consistency are combined with integrity and perseverance. Follow-through is the foundation of trust, and you must be the embodiment of this trait.

Family, friends, clients, peers, and community must trust you and see you as a resource, example, and vassal. That is correct, I believe in large part, we are the vassal or servant of our sphere of influence. This is one strategy to affect our external environments and solidify a support structure in our lives. When we strive to love ourselves, it is easier to meet the needs of others, and we expand beyond the limits of our perspective and internal issues.

By extending your passion and love to others, your own goal to improve habits transcends the confines of your mind and intrinsically supports your efforts. Again, the nature of life and the turbulence of external forces will batter and challenge the resolve of each individual.

Those with the enterprise to apply action to their passion will often meet greater resistance and confront more obstacles than those merely living life as a spectator or ignoring the destructive habits.

By increasing the opportunity for self-improvement and behavior change, we also gain greater exposure to challenges that will test our resolve or ability. However, the reward for those who place focused, passionate action towards a plan will reap intrinsic and potential extrinsic rewards that will far exceed the cost of failure or the pain of momentary obstacles.

The fear of things unknown or the taunting of failure may provoke paralysis or tempt perseverance to wane. To be implicit, I do not suggest a reckless plummet into the void of uncertainty but advocate the execution of a thoughtful and articulate plan that will serve as a guide for the application of passion.

Invest in your Personality

I believe as human beings; we each possess the capacity to actively improve our character. The desire to passionately improve is admirable but the pursuit of self-realization is about the elevation of conscious thought. Humans are unique in that we can mindfully pursue knowledge along with the means to apply wisdom derived from experience. This ability provides everyone the potential of improving personal behavior.

This realization enables human beings to manage responses and elevate social intelligence along with emotional sense. Our ability to adapt internal decision-making and temper emotional reflex grants the personal understanding needed to influence our responses and evolve our thought process. Our behaviors and response affect the way others regard us but more importantly, how we regard ourselves.

It is the eclectic collection of genetics, experiences, knowledge, and behavioral traits that collude to support our personality. The concept of self-improvement must be accepted if one is to maneuver life's challenges proactively with the mindset of a victor. The alternative is to admit weakness, place blame, and obstinately maintain the role of a victim. Become the change you desire internally, and the external results have a greater chance of manifesting accordingly.

When we carry a better understanding of ourselves and manage the quality of our internal speech, we may project positive energy to external persons within our sphere of connectivity and influence. This energy will affect family, friends, clients, coworkers, and any other human beings that enter the circle of your life.

Effective communication is also a byproduct of this positive internal thought process and a reasonable empathy towards other people's perspectives and thoughts will progress relationships and fortify trust. A quick note: I mentioned that personal perception is not a permeant reality, yet we must be able to see other perspectives so we can better communicate.

This is especially true if others in your sphere will not consider alternate perspectives, and the circumstances of your life require you to engage with them. Essentially, developing a personality rooted in consciousness, courtesy and compassion can dramatically improve relationships and the environment. The question becomes, what impression do you wish to leave within the hearts and minds of others and how will you use this power?

Navigate with Agility

To work towards our goals with a strong passion and improving personality, we must remain quite agile to avoid getting stuck or not recognizing when we may need to alter our projected plans. Specifically, when we lay out a strategy for any goal, we must identify any resistance to our efforts and be careful not to allow ego, stubbornness, or other negative traits to blind us from pitfalls.

This is not to say abandon determination, it simply means having an agile mind and being willing to make changes based on new information. Sometimes, we can allow our personal feelings about projects or goals to interfere with our rational decision-making processes and this can delay or destroy our purpose.

I see this quite often with entrepreneurs and small business owners I coach. I completely understand the deep emotional connection we can develop to our ideas, plans, brand, and businesses.

But obstinance and a stiff mind will certainly interfere with successful outcomes. In fitness and nutrition, I see many people get stuck with comfortable workout routines that become ineffective over time, make plans outside of their capacity, set unreasonable timeframes for goals, subscribe to dogmatic concepts, and not let go even when they do not see results.

We must remain agile and know when to make alterations to our plans or consider new ideas or approaches. When we put aside bias and consider alternative perspectives, we can add more tools to our resources, and this often facilitates more creativity and solution discovery. Closed minds are always married to a closed heart, so be nimble, open, and solution-oriented.

Develop Perseverance

People give up quickly with personal development, particularly habits related to fitness and nutrition management. Really damn quick indeed. I have observed two primary issues that stifle perseverance. First, we create arbitrary, unrealistic, or obscure goals that lack any true motivation. Sure, we want to lose weight or change an aspect of our habits but in the end, motivators must transcend aesthetics.

I can say with certainty; body composition is not a motivator for most people. While it is the most popular or desired outcome, it is not a strong long-term fuel and rarely a driver for perseverance. This is evident in the fact that we let ourselves get to a place where we are now seeking to change. We do not simply wake up one morning with an extra 80 lbs hanging from our bodies. This takes time to accumulate and body composition was compromised months or even years ago.

If our body composition or aesthetics were that important and a real motivator, we would have never even gained the weight, to begin with. Think about that. We allow ourselves to become unhealthy and over-fat through a period where dress sizes go up, trousers no longer fit, and our bodies degrade. But because the consequences are delayed and accumulate slowly, we can justify or ignore the negative change because the tradeoff seems more appealing.

The instant gratification from food or being lazy serves today and the consequences are minimal at the time. The process of accumulation proves that in the end, we pay the price. Second, we have unreasonable and even unrealistic expectations for return. Like I mentioned above, our desire for instant gratification and minimal effort hinders our prime motivators and our likelihood to persevere is diminished.

This is because perseverance, by its definition, is maintaining the resolve to do something despite difficulty or delay in achieving success. It's a long-term concept, and this conflicts with many of our societal conveniences and immediate gratification addictions. Perseverance is uniquely tied to passion, personality, and agility, which can determine the level of difficulty each individual may experience with perseverance.

Thankfully, we can initiate personal change and by finding our passion-based motivators and refining our personality consciously and deliberately, we can affect the change we desire. Now that we have this foundation, we can begin to hone our intelligent personality traits that comprise the power of our attraction and expose the opportunity for real habit alteration.

Chapter Keynotes

Taking ownership of our life and wellness is all about developing intended outcomes. We must recognize where we are in our physical and psychological state and identify if this is following our life plan. When we observe areas of our life that are antagonistic to our goals, we must adjust. Finding passion, investing in personal development, navigating with agility in our direction while persevering will help you F.I.N.D. your way.

- We must prioritize our personal development to affect our automated behavior, habit imprints, and improve conscious response.
- To some degree, the perception of others is fundamental to improving your external environment and because we do not live in a closed system, we must be aware of how we affect people in our circle.
- If you expect to be a person of reasonable influence and success who can develop their life outcomes, you must be willing to examine multiple perspectives and compare to your bias and see if there is room for you to modify and progress your mindset, which is a shift in perspective.
- Perception changes with information, time, environment, and experience. Therefore, all perception is temporary for those seeking self-improvement.
- Do not get attached to your perceptions or you will always be blinded, and it will be hard to F.I.N.D your way.
- Consider the four components of the F.I.N.D principle that drive your intended outcomes and set the stage for successfully improving your sphere of influence or external environment.
- **F = Focus on Your Passion:** There is no greater pursuit than passionately seeking to improve oneself.
- **I = Invest in Your Personality:** There is no greater challenge than the pursuit of self-realization.

- **N = Navigate with Agility:** There is no greater form of mental agility than minimizing personal bias or ego and discovering joy in the journey of personal development.
- **D = Develop Perseverance:** There is no greater source of self-affirmation than persevering and overcoming the most challenging obstacles.
- The power of a dynamic personality is simply that of attraction. When you focus on improving these areas, a natural byproduct is often an enhanced sense of self-love.
- When we love ourselves, we trust ourselves and the risk for relapse is reduced.
- Action is the kinetic component of change and evidence of true self-love.
- If we initiate personal improvement by finding our passion-based motivators and refining our personality consciously and deliberately we can affect the change, we desire.

"

AUTHORS PERSONAL NOTE

There are few things worse than a person with a terrible and unattractive personality. I develop my power of attraction because it magnetizes the best people towards me and repels those who would pollute my efforts to improve. Like-minded and strong personalities are incredibly supportive, but you have to attract them first by improving yours.

Chapter Eight
SEVEN INTELLIGENT PERSONALITY TRAITS

Self-love and internal respect are fundamental to behavior change. When we love ourselves, we will work hard to rectify areas in our lives we feel lack or are destructive, much as we will work to preserve high-value relationships with others. This means we need to work on our power of attraction and total contribution to improve our sphere of influence.

I use the word attraction outside of aesthetics and suggest it in terms of admiration. Self-admiration differs from narcissism. It is very appropriate to be proud of the positive traits you possess or have developed. Although the desirable character and personality profiles can be subjective and divergent by culture or society, I have developed a list of "Seven Intelligent Personality Traits" I affirm as fundamentally necessary for developing a well-rounded and captivating personality.

The point is, when we can influence our environments to some degree, we create that secondary support structure and this helps sustain our behavior objectives. The power of attraction reduces potential external risk because others will value their relationship with you and will seek to preserve it.

I struggled with the concept of naming the seven traits' "disciplines" over "intelligence" but decided that intelligence requires aptitude, reasoning, and accumulative capacity along with active mental and emotional management of information. This outline of the "Seven Intelligent Personality Traits" exemplifies the power of attraction, communication, and influence:

Intelligent Self-Awareness

In the simplest terms, self-awareness means you possess a clear picture of who you are or want to be. There is an understanding of personal strengths, weaknesses, biases, beliefs, desires, motivations, emotions, and perspectives. By grasping the tenants of your core character and thought process, you will have the power of alteration. Positive and value-based behavior modification is evidence of self-awareness.

Having the agility to alter reaction allows for personal growth and movement towards desired core character traits which improves your ability to project those changes. Knowing yourself and processing external stimulation by contrasting the input to your core character will challenge the strength of that character and conviction of self-trust. It is then a process of thoughtful comparisons that will provide options for behavior.

If our ethical and moral structure, prime motivators, or wellbeing are challenged, we instinctively react in the manner of our practiced core values. Therefore, we must seek to ingrain quality traits and bind them to our conscious selves. Over time and through consistent practice, these quality traits become subconscious and part of our unique manner of response. This is similar in principle to practicing physical skills found in athletics, playing instruments, or military maneuvers. Practice makes improvement.

Also, when we display consistency in behavior aligned with our speech, we create concord in our relationships and with ourselves. When we are intelligently self-aware, our behavior becomes consistent, and we project trustworthiness. When we are an example of emotional stability and steadfast resolve, we project an immensely powerful magnetism. Internal trust means you believe yourself and will be far more likely to adhere to your efforts toward habit change and maintain your fitness and nutrition objectives even during times of difficulty.

Intelligent Trust

Trust is the foundation of relationships, and this includes self-trust, which I submit is crucial for habit alteration and sustainability. I also see trust as a currency on which the economy of relationships either succeeds or fails. As I pointed out in Intelligent Self-Awareness when our words and behaviors align, we create consistency, and this fosters trust. Before we explore internal and external trust, let me illustrate the nature of trust. I like to think of trust as currency and each of us has a "trust account."

Like all banks, you can make deposits or withdrawals. If you make deposits, over time, you grow the balance into a positive surplus. However, mismanagement of trust will cause a withdrawal and eventually, an overdraft. Intelligent Trust is the deliberate act of making as many deposits as one can into their own internal account and the trust accounts of others, thus building tremendous equity.

Internal trust is when you believe you will do what you say. For example, if you set a goal of four workouts each week and you chronically skip, you start to make personal trust withdrawals. Over a short period, you no longer even believe yourself and have created a deficit in your personal account. I surmise the subconscious cannot distinguish the difference between you or an outside force eroding your personal trust.

To our minds, the withdrawal is made and deep down, you no longer trust yourself. We see evidence of this in reoccurring events such as lack of exercise adherence, poor food choices, abandoned diets, and so on.

To correct the overdraft, we must follow through with our plans and meet the commitments we set for ourselves. Every time you show up and work out, you make a deposit. Each day you stay on track with food, another deposit. Each day of doing what you said you would do in your career, at home, or with relationships adds more trust to your account.

Developing self-trust is necessary if you want to be an expert at financing others' trust. External trust is the value of accounts within your sphere of influence and is just as important as your account. When we make external deposits, we can further improve our power of attraction and solidify a remarkably strong support system.

One way I improved my self-trust was on the treadmill. I love outdoor walks and backcountry but dislike treadmills by comparison. You know, I will just say it...I hate doing indoor cardio. So, I used this as a game to build trust. I set a goal one winter to walk at least thirty minutes on a treadmill on scheduled days for one week. After that week of success and trust deposits, I committed to adding five minutes the following week to each walk. I met that commitment and moved the bar a little more.

Over four weeks, I got a full hour walk on scheduled days without fail. This is because I built my trust equity and knew I would follow through. Had I started at an hour, I feel I may not have been as successful, but the combination of progressive goals and execution developed my internal trust intelligently.

Intelligent Integrity

It is impossible to possess steady integrity without self-awareness and high equity trust accounts. Integrity is when you say what you mean with truth, and the language collaborates behavior.

If you have no connection to what you like, value, or believe you cannot form a solid moral basis because the lack of foundational concepts will not support the structure of integrity. If you do not have a personality supported by a type of morality, it will be challenging to compare or meet defined ethical standards in and out of wellness habits.

Do not be confused between the meaning of morals and ethics as it relates to integrity. Morals are an internal set of values or beliefs, whereas ethics are a set of externally accepted principles or rules. We tend to live by the edict of our morals but do so within the vein of an ethical standard.

Looking at the literal definition of integrity alone supports that statement. Integrity is a code of specific moral or artistic values or the state of being whole and undivided.

Your personality must be equally resolute, and a defining set of personal principles must be clear and expressed. We must be intelligent about the nature of integrity and ensure we satisfy our moral standards while meeting reasonable professional and social expectations. Maintaining one's integrity is crucial to the practice of consistency and is fundamental to trust within relationships, professional or social environments, and, most importantly, within ourselves.

I use integrity as a word to codify morals and ethics into a usable term specifically for objectively developing your personality and habits. I suggest you even write out your code of ethics. I have done this for Forge and have them posted on my website because they make up the backbone for decisions within my company. This has allowed me to create conscious action and build strong professional habits attuned to my integrity.

Intelligent Courage

Courage, by its definition, is the mental or moral strength to venture, persevere, and withstand danger, fear, or difficulty. It does not mean you do not feel fear, it means you can overcome it. One of the most paralyzing emotions we feel is fear in all levels of intensity. Over the years, I have seen so many people delay or stop their progress with better nutrition and activity because they were afraid.

The most common is the fear of starting a program and putting forth effort without seeing results. It's the fear of wasting time, energy, and even money that can derail wellness objectives. It is also the fear of change, even if the change is definitively for the better. We are indeed creatures of habit and are always looking for homeostasis even if that balance is negative.

Courage is a skill, and it takes a thoughtful reflection of what or why you are feeling fear to intelligently enhance your courage. It comes with acknowledging some likely uncomfortable aspects of your life and you must boldly address them. Courage ties back directly to passion, personality, agility, and perseverance.

In passion, we follow our convictions, and when we have that as a foundation, we are suited to act courageously. In personality, it is when we are afraid, yet consciously act to overcome that fear, and the very nature of action validates courage. Mental agility allows us to determine the total risk and adjust the course as we address our fear.

Courage is present in perseverance as beautifully displayed in Lord of The Rings, as the halflings Frodo and Sam struggle through Middle-earth to destroy the One Ring in the fires of Mount Doom. Despite their incredible fear and endless obstacles, they never give up and save the world through their courage and efforts.

Nothing worth doing is typically easy and we must face the challenges of life and our responses to it with intelligent courage. There is a significant difference between recklessness and courage, so be sure you are on the right side of it.

Intelligent Humor

Humor is not only a primary stress release mechanism; it is considered a deeply attractive trait. While many of us are born with an innate sense of humor, it is a skill you can improve. Of course, not all humor is the same, so we must maintain an intelligence about it. To clarify, I am not speaking specifically about comedy, which includes scripted television, stand-up, or media like that.

Having an open mind and reasonable tolerance for various types of humor can be helpful, but some manufactured stuff just isn't funny. More specifically, Intelligent humor is the breadth and depth of your capacity to find joy and levity in the general aspects of life and still know when to take things seriously. We have all met those folks who take things too seriously or worse, themselves.

On the flip side, some use humor with exceedingly poor timing. There is a time and place to be serious or use humor as a deflection, but it is not most of the time. This is where intelligence comes in. In habit alteration, humor can be a helpful trait to keep a positive perspective and disallow negative thoughts and feelings.

Intelligent Emotional Sense

Having a highly tuned emotional sense allows you to assess your reactions and assists in the Power of Conscious Response. The ability to pause the automation of your emotional reactions will allow you to delay or alter reception and develop a response in line with your intended outcome. Because many of our instigators stem from emotions, having a strong intelligence about our sensitivities gives us more control. Or at least, allows us to be better stewards of our attitudes.

Learning to objectively assess emotional response and comparing it to the instigator before a reaction can be immensely helpful. Often, we will allow our typical automated response to activate without that assessment and find ourselves in a situation where we overreact, make a poor choice, or do not behave in a manner aligned with our intention. Taking a moment to decide how to respond is a practice in active consciousness and patience.

Developing a heightened emotional sense is certainly a skill and one worth taking time and energy to improve. It translates to keeping calm under pressure, better decision making, less regretful reactions, and an elevated feeling of personal control. Progressing your emotional sense also nicely translates to improved professional and personal relationships. By slowing the response from instigators, you may better prepare your reactions in multiple environments.

Remember, your feelings are like perceptions, and we should be careful how much stock we place in them. Often, I see people respond in a negative and overdramatic way to what appears to be a relatively mild or insignificant situation. But by their response, you would think the world is ending. After a period in which they completely embarrass themselves with their behavior, they step back and realize their emotional reaction was unjustified and now they must make the apology tour.

This is where someone who mismanaged their emotional state must go around the office or the house apologizing for the outburst and overreaction. Be selective about where you put your emotional energy and consider what your perspective may be after the incident that raises your ire has passed. I like to jump ten minutes ahead in my mind and try to project how I will feel after the incident has passed.

Nearly every single time I think about my emotional response before reacting, I make a much better choice in reply posture, tone, words used, and so on. One note on emotional sense and social media: I think that these platforms are a perversion of social interaction and allow people to be just awful to each other without repercussion. I have seen people emotionally engaging with each other in negative, highly explicit, or inappropriate ways and this is a disgrace.

I encourage you to avoid using social media for personal or political debate or make emotional reactions as it is counterproductive and serves no value and kills emotional sense. Your angry partisan rebuttal to a political meme is not changing the world one bit, but it sure is making your life miserable.

Intelligent Discipline

Often, folks struggling with their fitness or food-management are criticized for a lack of discipline. While this may be the case for some, lack of discipline is not always the primary factor, but it certainly is a contributor.

Usually, our inability to successfully identify and alter bad habits override any potential discipline. We can only apply the skill of discipline if we understand the nature of our current condition and have a projected outcome to which we may apply a set of defined practices.

Another challenge with discipline is the cyclical nature of many of our efforts. For example, we may be able to assert a significant amount of temporary discipline towards a goal for a period, but it will falter over time as motivation wanes. Intelligent discipline is the ability to link our efforts and motivators to an outcome for sustainability and recognize that we can improve our Intelligent Discipline like any skill we practice.

Even highly tuned discipline may not be linear and having a plan in place that allows for breaks or undulation of effort will add to the longevity of your intention. We often use the words self-control and discipline interchangeably, but really, we are talking about a code of behavior to which we are trying to adhere.

Our intelligent discipline must be based on a defined set of preventive strategies, supportive actions, and a system for correction or reward. The very nature of our set discipline must be rooted in positive reinforcement and uplifting self-talk. Personal punishment or self-flagellation is destructive and not intelligent discipline, so be sure you base this strategy on high positivity and objective review.

Chapter Keynotes

The power of attraction is not always an aesthetic, it includes the value of your character and esteem. Those who practice self-love and work to improve their core personality can not only improve their responses to instigators but also attract a great deal of support.

- We must prioritize our personal development to affect our automated behavior and hopefully, influence the dynamics of our external environments.
- When we love ourselves, we will work hard to rectify areas in our lives we feel lack or are destructive, much as we will work to preserve high-value relationships with others.
- **Intelligent Self-Awareness** means one has a clear picture of their strengths, weaknesses, bias, beliefs, desires, motivations, emotions, and perspectives.
- Knowing yourself and processing external stimulation by contrasting the input to core character will challenge the strength of that character and conviction of self-trust.
- When we display consistency in behavior aligned with our speech, we create concord in our relationships and with ourselves. When we are intelligently self-aware, our behavior becomes consistent, and we project trustworthiness.
- **Intelligent Trust** is the currency on which the economy of relationships either succeeds or fails.
- Intelligent Trust is the deliberate act of making as many deposits as one can into their internal account and the trust accounts of others, thus building tremendous equity.
- It seems the subconscious cannot distinguish the difference between you or an outside force eroding your personal trust.
- Every time you show up and workout, you make a deposit. Each day you stay on track with food, another deposit. Each day of doing what you said you would do in your

career, at home, or with relationships adds more trust to your account.

- When we make internal and external deposits of trust, we can further improve our power of attraction and solidify a remarkably strong support system.
- **Intelligent Integrity** is when you say what you mean with truth, and the language collaborates behavior.
- Morals are an internal set of values or beliefs, whereas ethics are a set of externally accepted principles or rules.
- Integrity is a code of specific moral or artistic values or the state of being whole and undivided.
- Maintaining one's integrity is crucial to the practice of consistency and is fundamental to trust within relationships, professional or social environments, and, most importantly, within ourselves.
- **Intelligent Courage** is the mental or moral strength to venture, persevere, and withstand danger, fear, or difficulty.
- Courage is a skill, and it takes a thoughtful reflection of what or why you are feeling fear to intelligently enhance your courage.
- Mental agility allows us to determine the total risk and adjust the course as we address our fear.
- Nothing worth doing is typically easy and we must face the challenges of life and our responses to it with intelligent courage.
- **Intelligent Humor** is the breadth and depth of your capacity to find joy and levity in the general aspects of life and still know when to take things seriously.
- In habit alteration, humor can be a helpful trait to keep a positive perspective and disallow negative thoughts and feelings.
- **Intelligent Emotional Sense** allows you to assess your reactions and assists in the Power of Conscious Response.
- Because many of our instigator's stem from emotions, having a strong intelligence about our sensitivities gives us

more control. Or at least, allows us to be better stewards of our attitudes.

- Intelligent emotional sense translates to keeping calm under pressure, better decision making, less regretful reactions, and an elevated feeling of personal control.
- I encourage you to never use social media for personal debate or make emotional reactions as it is counterproductive and serves no value and kills emotional sense.
- **Intelligence Discipline** is understanding the nature of our current condition and has a projected outcome to which we may apply a set of defined practices.
- Even highly tuned discipline may not be linear and having a plan in place that allows for breaks or undulation of effort will add to the longevity of your intention.
- Our intelligent discipline must be based on a defined set of preventive strategies, supportive actions, and a system for correction or reward.
- Discipline bridges the gap between low levels or fluctuations of motivation towards your goals.

"

I am never afraid to set incredibly ambitious goals because I intended to succeed and find joy in the effort. The mountain top provides beautiful views but do not forget to enjoy the lakes, rivers, trees, and wildlife on the path to the summit. Sometimes, the journey is equally valuable as the destination.

Chapter Nine
SETTING REALISTIC EXPECTATIONS AND GOALS

Setting realistic expectations is a necessary step to maintaining momentum and provides an objective system for measuring progress. Establishing boundaries assists with the keeping of internal promises and can mitigate potential external instigators. I like to combine setting expectations with boundaries because they define the potential outcome and demark the playing field of life. Let's look at the steps for setting both reasonable expectations and establishing boundaries.

Setting Expectations

Too often, I see folks setting unreasonable expectations between their envisioned outcome, willingness, and genetic predisposition. When we create goals or expectations that are over-hard or nearly impossible, we do not set ourselves up for sustainable success. Instead, we become bitter, discouraged, and sink back into the cycle of fitness failure. When we envision an outcome, we must be certain it is within our scope or capacity and is a genetic possibility.

I have worked with a young woman who is now in college that started with me when she was a sophomore in high school. I have watched her mature and learn so much about how to create her unique style of fitness despite her incredible study workload and the distractions of youth.

A few years back, she sent me a series of screenshots featuring Instagram models and incredibly genetically gifted women. Her caption in the message said something to the effect of "this is where I want to get my body." While I can appreciate looking at physiques for inspiration or ideas on how to improve personal aesthetics, we must be objective about our potential.

This young woman stands at about five-foot flat, with more of an endomorphic disposition, has always struggled with excess body fat, is on hormone therapy, and has only a few hours each week she can commit to structured exercise. The models she used for example stand well over five foot ten, have mesomorphic advantages, surgical alterations, and a tremendous amount of time dedicated to exercise.

As I stated earlier, most of these "models" are paid by supplement and product companies to exercise as much as possible and sell their products. Essentially, these are professional exercisers and advertisers, so they have the time and motivation to dedicate themselves.

Anyhow, looking at these pictures, I knew instantly the likelihood of her achieving this outcome would be slim at best. I also knew that despite how uncomfortable the conversation was, I would have to help her understand her likely potential and still coach her through the disappointment and move towards reasonable expectations.

Let's explore why her expectations or goal of high-level aesthetics were unrealistic and then talk about how to make the attitude shift towards reality. First, her height and somatotype would be the first incredible obstacle to overcome. As an endomorph, she would have to ensure her food was completely on target and her exercises would need to be specific and intense.

But even if she could move the needle for a time into some aspects of mesomorphic proportion, she could not sustain it forever. To compound this, she was in a dorm with limited cooking capacity, and the university food court dealt mostly with low nutrition, processed, and pre-packaged foods. Second, her study and class schedule presented a major obstacle of available time, and she would not be able to put in the hours each week necessary to signal that level of adaptation in the body.

Finally, her willingness to focus so intensely on what would be required was simply not there. At the time, she had no concept of what it would take but knew it would require more than she was currently doing. This presented me with several problems to solve and the pressure to make a positive out of a disappointing reality was tough. In the end, I went to my trusty standby of direct honesty.

On our next coaching call, I decided to explain what would be required for her to achieve anything close to her imagined outcome. I was careful to highlight the beauty of our potential and to make this the cornerstone of our goal setting.

However, I also explained the reality behind somatotype and that I suspected she was firmly in the realm of endomorphic and her height would dictate much of the aesthetic differences between what she saw in her head versus what was reasonable, plus the copious amounts of elective surgical enhancements required.

Like most people who hear bad news, she had an emotional response to it. After a time, she wiped away the tears and asked, "So what you are saying is that I will never look like this no matter how hard I try?" To which I responded, "You will never look exactly like any of these models you showed me. They have over ten inches of height on you, genetic advantage, time, willingness, massive structural support, and surgical embellishment. For your wellbeing, we need to discover what is reasonable and sustainable for you and decide how close you are willing to get to your unique genetic potential and find joy there."

I refuse to feed my clients popular lies about what is reasonable and it's about damn time people be realistic with their goal setting in fitness. Needless suffering, dissatisfaction, and unhappiness stemming from unreasonable physical comparisons are so destructive and a terrible emotional trap.

This is why I never use before-and-after images of clients in any marketing for Forge. It's so disingenuous and makes false comparisons. Enabling unrealistic and overly superficial desires are the opposite of what I want to accomplish as a professional. Compare yourself to yourself, not the over-filtered professional models you see in the media.

One of the best ways to set reasonable expectations for yourself is to acknowledge a few key points. First, we need to determine our somatotype and then look for all the advantages and potential our genetics provide. Do not focus on the negative aspects of your body or base physiological make-up. It is counterproductive and cannot be fundamentally changed, so leave it alone and change your attitude about it. When in doubt, go back to the 30x3+10 rule.

I always wanted a Capitan America body, but I was given a Spiderman physique and have resolved to love it and make it the best I can. Second, once you have determined your likely genetic potential, you must decide to what degree you are willing to put in the work to get close to that potential. If life circumstances only present a certain level of opportunity for exercise, then maximize it.

Third, once you get to your genetic potential or to whatever level is reasonable, you must be happy with the results. Find joy in your own body and only compare to your alternative self. Of course, admiring others is fine, but admiration is a long way from coveting and idolizing others for things that are not and cannot be yours. You may only get to 70% of your potential but if that is all you are willing to do, then your joy must still be 100%.

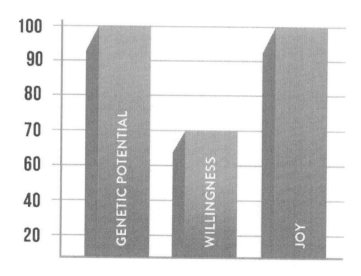

The Motivation Myth

When considering our expectations and goals, we must clearly define why and how we intend to start, measure, and meet our objectives. While we certainly can outline intrinsic and extrinsic motivators, these are rarely sustaining because inspiration without habit-based behavior change will likely end in lost momentum.

This is because motivation is an emotion and like all emotions, subject to change. I find this to be especially true with fitness goals because of the long-term nature and delayed reward. It is often helpful to break goals down into milestones to allow for more frequent achievement.

However, we must be careful not to become addicted to the feeling of motivation because this inevitably leads to procrastination or lost interest. By aligning our habit behaviors toward a particular goal, we create an action potential. It is the structure of these behaviors that deliver results, not motivation.

Of course, motivation plays an important role in the process of getting started or setting goals, but it has limited usefulness thereafter. There will be days you simply do not "feel like it" because of the inevitability of impeding factors. It can be as simple as weather changes, lack of sleep, or personal and professional distractions, or competing emotions that change how you feel about your goal and the assessment of effort.

This is dangerous because we are tying an emotional catalyst to our goal instead of changing our habits, which can breed procrastination. When this happens, we start saying things like "I really don't feel motivated to do my workout" or "I am feeling so demotivated right now."

When we expect to have a constant flow of motivation to take action, we forfeit our power to progress because we are now relying on emotion instead of conscious discipline. If this happens, we set ourselves up for frustration or discouragement. We must not allow our constantly changing emotional state to dictate our behaviors toward goals or rely on surges of fleeting motivation.

Exercise and food management are for a lifetime, and it is unreasonable to assume you will always be motivated. But in the end, success comes from doing it anyway. Real progress comes from doing what you set out to do long after the inspiration to do it has fled.

Instead, it is Intelligent Discipline that we need to foster because discipline is a skill. The days or moments we don't "feel motivated" are precisely when we need to execute that discipline. Like all skills, it must be practiced, and the more you do practice, the higher your adherence to the efforts that lead to your objective.

In addition, the disciplined follow-through on behaviors needed to achieve a milestone or goal intrinsically reinforce habit development and often reduce the frequency of destructive motivation loss.

Limiting Beliefs

Each day, we are forced to deal with and guide our thoughts through endless levels of limiting or negative self-talk and belief. We must work against our self-imposed limitations and overcome personal fear, doubt, or negative internal conversations about our situations or progress toward goals. To remove a limiting belief, we must proactively take charge of our repeated thoughts and internal affirmations. Be it positive or negative, we slowly believe at a subconscious level what we say consciously.

Strive to uncover your limiting beliefs and expose them so you may create strategies to remove them. I encourage you to avoid identifying with those ideas or manufactured beliefs that limit your ability to exceed your status. Question your conclusions and never concede the energy from negative thoughts regarding your ability or potential as truth. Test and challenge your perceptions and become active in your responses and be the change internally so the external benefits may follow.

If you believe you will fail before you start, then you create a self-fulfilling prophecy and will likely do just that. Be certain not to confuse limiting beliefs with unrealistic expectations as we must have attainable goals. If your objectives are realistic, then nothing should stand in your way, especially yourself.

5 Steps for Setting Goals

Follow these five simple steps to creating a set of reasonable expectations for yourself based on a realistic assessment with your personal potential as the focal point:

Specify Your Goals

Goal setting is a powerful and necessary aspect of developing intended outcomes and serves as a system for checking progress. We must be specific with our goal setting and align as many intrinsic values as possible to each goal. Extrinsic goals are fine, but we need to ensure maximal motivational ties are associated with what we are trying to accomplish. I have found many people make ambiguous goals based on a superficial outcome, but these are rarely powerful enough to maintain motivation.

Yes, I have seen some people successfully set an aesthetic goal and be quite successful, but in general, we need to dig deeper if we plan on sustaining our wellness. In the 90-Day Habit Transformation workbook, you can address your motivators and align specific and strategic goals to each motivator to jump-start your enthusiasm for accomplishment.

Specifying your goals will assist in creating the task list of things you must do to meet your goal. Without specifics, you cannot formulate a coherent plan with realistic and measurable action items that lead to success. Recently I worked with a young man through the 90-Day Habit Transformation program and after completing that, he moved over to one of my regular coaching programs for maintenance, so I have come to know him well.

One of his biggest challenges initially was setting specific goals. He struggled to figure out precisely what he wanted. In the workbook, his answers were initially vague and incomplete. He was invested in the program and was taking actionable steps but just could not seem to quantify his desired outcome with specificity. He was able to set one specific goal, but even that was relatively vague because the process of achievement had so many variables.

After the 90-Day program, I had him go back and complete the workbook all over again to see if the journey uncovered more of his personal consciousness. Nearly every time I have a client go through the workbook again at the end of the program, their answers are far more detailed, specific, and aligned to their life plan. In this second round, he identified nearly a half-dozen specific goals and tied them directly to his intended outcome.

He set aside limiting beliefs and identified his motivations, instigators and elevated his wellness consciousness. Armed with this awareness, he was able to better articulate and specify what he wanted for himself, his career, and his family. He became specific with his goal-setting but that was after he took the time for self-improvement and discovery. Know thy self.

Be Realistic

Goals and intended outcomes should be objectively scrutinized to ensure you are working towards a realistic result. Too often, we think of our goals in terms of the final result and fail to see the critical waypoints towards achievement. Playing towards a long-term objective is great but set short-term goals that support your overall life design. It is also important that your goals be possible and set with a strong objective mindset.

Setting goals that are not realistic will certainly cause frustration and eventual disappointment. If you are not capable or it is genetically impossible to achieve a goal, then do not set it. Likewise, do not set goals you know deep down you will not work towards. Occasionally, I have observed clients setting goals they know they cannot achieve.

I call this "leaving an exit." Sadly, people will self-sabotage their potential right from the start by setting unrealistic goals. That way, when working towards them, they can always bail out citing it's too hard, unrealistic, or whatever excuse they can conjure to justify quitting.

If you have no desire to run a marathon and lack attachment to the journey and outcome, don't set that as a goal. This is because, in your case, the process is not equal to or greater than the reward.

I want to clarify that what may be a realistic goal for someone else may not be a realistic goal for yourself. Oh, sure, you may be physically capable, but if you are not psychologically willing, then the body will not follow.

Sometimes we need to set goals that are not necessarily exciting but have a big realistic or tangible payoff. For example, I have a client who is always looking for some kind of new approach to keep his workouts fresh.

We have done incline challenges, push-up, and pull-up challenges, 5k's, 10k's, and half marathons just to name a few. During one of our coaching sessions, we were discussing some new ideas to create some measurable adaptations and keep things interesting.

This client has had a highly active life and over time accumulated some mobility issues and biomechanical malalignments, particularly in the shoulders and neck. I have been trying to get him to add in some corrective work for years, but he never really got into it and was resistant.

With some encouragement which he playfully called nagging, he decided it was finally time to address this issue, and even though postural and mobility workouts are famously dull, he set the goal of improving his biomechanical function and bearing.

I built him a specialized corrective exercise program to help reduce the excessive protraction of the shoulders and forward jutting of the head. We set a goal of executing the "super boring" corrective workouts at least four times each week and scheduled them.

He was not enthusiastic about the exercises but understood that his mobility issues were impeding his potential, and his posture was the gateway to higher levels of fitness. Even though he was not overly excited about the corrective goal, he stuck with it and made significant progress in his posture in just a few months.

As a result, he greatly reduced his shoulder pain, headache frequency and progressed his lifting capacity with better biomechanical alignment. The point is the goal was not exciting on the surface, but the payoff from addressing his posture paid dividends. The goal was not unrealistic, it was just unappealing, and the process was monotonous, but with the right attitude became a worthwhile focus.

Interestingly, this client is now a huge advocate of corrective work, and we incorporate postural maintenance into all his programming. Just because a goal is not over-the-top exciting, does not mean it does not have a compelling purpose.

Be careful not to classify a goal as unrealistic just because you don't want to do it. But do not be afraid to set and embrace goals that are uncomfortable or not necessarily exciting provided there is that payoff.

On the other hand, if your goal is to have a twenty-foot vertical jump, then that is where you need to adjust for reality.

Set Plausible Timeframes

One mentor once said, "Your goals are likely not unrealistic, but the timeframe you set for those goals may be." I found this to be an encouraging yet cautionary perspective. After all, typical goal achievement is simply the execution of tasks focused on the realization of an intended outcome within a defined time.

We specify what we are trying to accomplish, take actionable steps to move that direction, and through consistent and agile applications meet that target. Simple. Except it's simple, just not easy.

We must learn to avoid setting unrealistic expectations, and this includes timeframes for achievement. The most common mistake people make with fitness and nutrition goal setting is the timeframe and return expectation for results.

I have mentioned it on several occasions throughout this book, but here it is again: You don't gain twenty pounds of fat in a week, and you most certainly will not lose it in that amount of time.

Without question, one of many major problems with most weight loss or diets is the overemphasis on the speed of loss and not the quality or sustainability. People are perfectly fine stuffing their faces and sitting on their butts all day for months or years.

But when they randomly or seasonally want to lose weight or "get healthy" they expect instant results with the least amount of effort and then get upset that it's not working overnight. Insert eye roll here.

I deal with this timeframe issue so much I did a little two-phase experiment in 2019 and shared the results openly with my clients. I spent twelve weeks abandoning exercise and eating like a typical American.

For example, this meant lowering my activity levels and instead of ordering salmon, brown rice, and asparagus, I would order a burger and perhaps a beer. The goal was to go twelve weeks like this to see what the effect on my composition and lifestyle would be.

The second phase was to spend another twelve weeks trying to get back to my initial starting stats and compare. Well, phase one lasted ten weeks because I could not take the damage any longer and began to experience definitive adverse effects.

My composition went foul, and my energy levels plummeted along with my mood. I experienced even more insomnia, and my skin even broke out in places, so I cut it two weeks short.

I started the experiment on July 29th, 2019, and by October 7th, 2019, I had gained 19 lbs of body fat, which was an 11.3% increase over my starting percentage. My lean muscle fell 8.2 lbs over the ten weeks as well. In phase two, my goal was to see how close I could get to my starting statistics within the same timeframe.

The trick is, I would bring all my expertise and discipline to bear and completely dial in for those ten recovery weeks. I wanted to see if I could revert within the same time it took to destroy. Nope. Not even with intense and highly structured exercise and precise nutrition could I make that happen.

While I made considerable improvement, I could not get back to the same fitness in an identical time frame. From October 8th, 2019, through December 15th, 2019, I was only able to reduce my body fat by 8.2%, leaving 3.1% to go until I got back to where I started.

The upside for me in the recovery came from developing lean muscle tissue because I was hyper-focused on progressive strength training. I rehabilitated nearly 11 lbs of muscle over the 10 recovery weeks so my weight stayed about the same between the initial and final weigh-in. As a side note, this is a perfect example of why I do not focus too much on cumulative body weight as it is an incomplete picture.

Anyway, I could not get my body fat back to the original percentage until my check-in on January 24th, 2020. It took nearly sixteen weeks from October of 2019 until January of 2020 for a professional trainer with a highly specific program to recover what was damaged in just ten weeks.

Let that sink in a little. It took sixteen weeks without a single mistake to fix something that took ten weeks to recklessly break without effort.

Now imagine, you do not have a specific exercise plan, handle on your nutrition and positive attitude about reasonable results. How long will it take to hit your goal and how sustainable will it be?

A final note related to timeframes and goals. A major stumbling block can be self-inflicted procrastination, which will mess with our timetables. I have two recommendations for overcoming procrastination.

First, write a list of all the tasks you must complete personally and professionally in order of easy to hardest. Then, attack all the items on this list that can be done immediately or within a few days of writing your list to get some momentum.

In this scenario, we do not prioritize, as this can create paralysis. It seems most of our procrastination can be related to complex or critical tasks, which may be time-consuming or unpleasant.

Sometimes prioritizing creates an additional problem as we become overwhelmed and the list seems insurmountable, and we continue procrastinating on the whole list. But if we can just get started and cross some items off that list, we are likely to take that forward progress and continue working through the tasks till completion.

The second method is the traditional approach of laying out all your tasks and prioritizing those which need immediate attention or the most important. By acknowledging and listing out tasks by order of importance, you can formulate a strategy to get it all done.

This lets you get the big stress items off your list as soon as possible so you can turn your attention to the remaining simple tasks. Your personality and mindset may be a major factor in which approach you choose.

Remember, you can always change how you address your task list, so do not get stuck in analysis paralysis. Now that we have a defined system for accomplishing tasks related to our goals, we can attach timeframes that are reasonable and set hard dates for completion.

I like to use an electronic calendar system for managing my workflow, events, tasks, and goals. They are usually all interconnected, so managing this way is easy for me.

You can also use a paper calendar, whiteboard, or anything that works for you and allows for proper management of your tasks. Calendars are a great way to manage tasks and goals because the visualization of time helps you manage procrastination. It also gives a sense of accomplishment when you can strike out or check off a task or goal as completed.

Measure Frequently

I have heard it said that what gets measured gets managed. Yes, indeed, this is true, but let's break this into three distinct stumbling blocks to avoid.

One, there is a significant difference between disciplined and obsessive tracking. Two, ignoring or avoiding the measurement of progress out of fear will not help you. Third, measuring and collecting data but not using it to alter your efforts or program will make the data useless. Now let's unpack these three issues.

Obsession vs Discipline

Tracking your fitness activities and food intake can be a positive and proactive form of self-management. Yet there is a definitive line between needless obsession and a disciplined lifestyle.

One of my long-time clients and amazing human named Danielle, wrote out her viewpoint as it relates to this topic, and I think it well articulated: "Discipline is self-control. When we make changes to live a healthier life, we will need a good amount of self-control to keep us on course.

We will likely need plans, both for meals and workouts, so we know how to stay on track and measure what is working. We must exercise restraint to stick to those goals when eating. We will need the fortitude to keep showing up to work out, even when tired or not in the mood.

Being consistent even when we don't want to be is self-discipline. Obsession is completely different. Obsession is a persistent preoccupation with achieving your goals or living your life a certain way.

When you are obsessed, your focus becomes your life. In terms of fitness, your attempt to be healthy can place unreasonable expectations on yourself.

It will most likely affect the other people in your life, placing unfair expectations on them as well. Obsession disrupts a healthy, balanced life. Instead of making healthy choices, your obsession runs your life."

As she points out, obsession is disruptive and manufacturers unnecessary stress and even resentment towards the process. A final note on this is about the issue I shared in earlier chapters related to my dissatisfaction with a genetic predisposition. As you may recall from a previous chapter, from 2012 until late 2015, I became obsessed with meeting my genetic potential.

Because my expectations were quite unrealistic, measurements became a constant obsession. I could never get my body to the level I was demanding and paid an emotional and physical toll.

Be sure your measurements are meant to help pursue disciplined goals that are realistic and within plausible timeframes. Trust me; it will save you pain and keep you from resenting fitness.

Measurement Avoidance

This may be one of the most common issues I must coach clients through related to goal setting and measurement. I would say a fair percentage of new clients find ways to avoid both initial measurements and progress evaluation.

Often, a client will refuse to take their body weight, circumference measurements, or photos because they fear the results. This is the mental equivalent of burying your head in the sand.

If you don't know where you started, it's hard to know where you are going and validate the direction. I also see this in the avoidance of calorie counting or meal planning. Occasionally, I work with a client that has a low-level or clinically disordered eating challenge.

If directed by a medical or mental health professional, it may be wise to avoid some methods of tracking because it can reinforce an eating disorder.

Unless that is the case in your situation, I highly recommend some method of tracking and measuring fitness and nutrition efforts. Avoiding a measurement just because you don't like the results is not a cause to ignore the value of information. Set your shame aside and measure what is important so you can manage your efforts and validate goal achievement.

Using Collected Data

Compared to the folks that avoid tracking, this group is not as large in general but enough to point it out. Engineers and mechanically minded clients tend to collect so much data it can be overwhelming.

Unfortunately, most of this data is wasted or needless. Another challenge I often see with folks that hoard data is they don't act on the information.

They can outline their hydration schedule, cumulative caloric output for the past week, and their precise macronutrient intake, but they get stuck there.

I have even worked with clients that use multiple tracking applications and consolidate all their data and graph it in a spreadsheet. My typical response is "Great! Now what?" This is where they stare blankly and slowly shrug their shoulders.

I am a huge fan of wearable technologies that support an active lifestyle and provide data. But this data must be relevant and usable. At a minimum, I recommend looking at your total activity output and food intake to simply compare to your objective.

We can get granular if that's what is needed, but in general, it's just a waste of time and energy to track every single detail if you don't use it.

One of my 90-Day Habit clients uses a very detail-oriented fitness tracker that loads all your data into a web application. You can sort and see just about every activity and trend. He had so much data and did not even know how to read most of it, so we went through it together.

We discovered some interesting energy readings we were able to associate with exercises and life events. It became clear that certain activities were not optimal for him compared to others. In his case, he goes to a high-intensity style workout three times each week and has been for many years.

We looked at the workouts for each day and compared them to his output. We concluded that his body had created a strong adaptation to the repetitive nature of his workouts and indicated a plateau in his progress.

We altered his workout variables and restructured his workout approach to send new stress and adaptation signals. That did the trick, and he broke the stale return on his efforts. We could validate with his fitness tracker that his output and physiological response improved with the changes. The point is having data is great, but you must be able to use it.

Goal Evaluation

Taking the time to evaluate goals for both potency and progress should be prioritized. As we explored with the F.I.N.D principle, we must have agility while on our journey.

Evaluation of our goals and the validity they hold in our intended outcomes can be intuitive or structured. I tend to like my goal evaluations loosely scheduled so I can be more deliberate in my planning and actions.

This is because many of my personal and professional goals are quite specific, so it's relatively easy to framework evaluation and schedule a progress review. However, there is something to be said about just knowing when and what to change based on your observations and instinct.

Regardless, we must take a measure of our progress and determine if we are on the right path, need to make minor course corrections, or even eliminate a goal.

Evaluation of a goal value is made simple by being specific and realistic from the beginning with a plausible scope and timeframe. Measuring frequently and using that data will help you determine the quality of each goal and makes evaluation manageable.

Chapter Keynotes

Setting realistic goals and expectations is a necessary aspect of habit alteration and personal success. We must be objective about what is reasonable and apply the correct behavior to achieve an outcome. We must also be very careful about setting time frames for goals to avoid needless discouragement and loss of motivation.

- When we set goals or expectations that are over-hard or nearly impossible, we do not set ourselves up for sustainable success.
- When we envision an outcome, we must be certain it is within our scope or capacity and is a genetic possibility.
- For your mental wellbeing, we need to discover what is reasonable and sustainable for your fitness outcome and decide how close you are willing to get to your unique genetic potential and find joy there.
- Needless suffering, dissatisfaction, and unhappiness stemming from unreasonable physical comparisons are so destructive and a terrible emotional trap.
- We must work against our own self-imposed limitations and overcome personal fear, doubt, or negative internal conversations about our situations or progress toward goals.
- We must all strive to uncover our limiting beliefs and expose them so we may create strategies to remove them.
- Question your conclusions and never concede the energy from negative thoughts regarding your ability or potential as truth.
- We must be specific with our goal setting and align as many intrinsic values as possible to each goal.
- Setting goals that are not realistic will certainly cause frustration and eventual disappointment.
- Just because a goal is not over-the-top exciting, does not mean it does not have a compelling purpose.

- Typical goal achievement is simply the execution of tasks focused on the realization of an intended outcome within a defined time.
- Your goals are likely not unrealistic, but the timeframe you set for those goals may be.
- Beware of procrastination or convoluting your goals.
- There is a definitive line between needless obsession and a disciplined goal-oriented lifestyle.
- Obsession is disruptive and manufacturers unnecessary stress and even resentment towards the process.
- Avoiding a measurement related to progress toward a goal just because you may not like the results is not a cause to ignore the value of information.
- we must be careful not to become addicted to the feeling of motivation because this inevitably leads to procrastination or lost interest.
- When we expect to have a constant flow of motivation to take action, we forfeit our power to progress because we are now relying on emotion instead of driven behavior.
- Real progress comes from doing what you set out to do long after the inspiration to do it has fled.
- Following through on the behaviors needed to achieve that milestone or goal intrinsically reinforce habit development and often reduce the frequency of destructive motivation loss.
- Taking the time to evaluate goals for both potency and progress should be prioritized.
- Evaluation of a goal value is made simple by being specific and realistic from the beginning with a plausible scope and timeframe.

66

AUTHORS PERSONAL NOTE

I learned boundaries start from within and once you know what you are willing to do or not do, the rest is just honest, loving communication.

Chapter Ten
SETTING PERSONAL AND PROFESSIONAL BOUNDARIES

Boundaries are essential for internal conversations or personal action and critical for managing external environments. Internally, boundaries help us adhere to our values, physical and emotional wellbeing, and maintain our self-identity.

Externally, boundaries help us communicate what is or is not acceptable behavior from others and help define our environments. This is a complex subject and for this book, we will only focus on boundary concepts that support habit alteration related to fitness and nutrition.

Let's explore how we can create and maintain personal and professional boundaries to support our efforts towards developing a habit. The foundation of boundaries is similar in both circumstances and includes your emotional value, physical value, and social value.

In clinical psychology, practitioners typically include intellectual and spiritual worth across the spectrum of human dynamics, but we will focus on the first three.

Psychologists further define boundaries by type such as healthy, rigid, or porous, but I am going to just give some tips and you can decide how to set your limits.

I have observed the best boundaries are set and adhered to by using a simple system of defining the boundary, communicating it without over-explanation, and expressing why it is important.

One arching theme is that boundaries are not just for others, they are also for yourself. Before we get into boundaries, let's review an interesting phenomenon of false priority and the lack of boundaries we set for our wellness.

A challenge many of us face is the tendency to separate our well-being from our system of prioritization in our professional and personal life.

We tend to break fitness and nutrition into separate categories and make them abstract concepts we revisit from time to time. It is quite common for people to manufacture these unnecessary compartments but do not confuse these damaging silos with supportive boundaries. We often put fitness in a silo and nutrition in another as a means of avoidance.

This means that someone may go on some type of diet but will neglect activity or structured fitness. On the other hand, people will start a workout program but do little in curbing their poor nutritional intake. This is because many of us do not see fitness and nutrition as equal parts of a wellness equation.

I see how this can happen because we do this in our personal and professional lives when we break out our personality traits into fragments and then compartmentalize. While a professional demeanor, behavior, and conversational content should be managed in the workplace, we are still the same person but metered to situations.

We most certainly must audit and censor ourselves in these environments or social dynamics and that makes perfect sense. However, there is no reason or benefit for separating fitness and nutrition and pretending it is unimportant.

We need to make wellness inclusive to every aspect of our lives, personally and professionally. This is precisely why we need to set specific boundaries in both environments. But the boundaries should not be at the expense of excluding wellness, it should be seamlessly integrated into your lifestyle and translate to personal and professional dynamics.

You cannot take care of your responsibilities optimally if you are unwell. It makes absolutely no sense to neglect your fitness and food choices at the expense of your wellbeing to satisfy a career or personal demand.

I often hear excuses about priority, time, energy, environment, and so on, but in the end, it's just an excuse. I know that's tough to hear but failing to set boundaries that support your wellbeing is counterproductive in any metric.

If your career choice or work environment routinely required you to sacrifice your health for deadlines or productivity, you may want to reconsider your choices.

Conversely, if you create a personal environment where your needs are met last or not at all, I recommend you strongly reconsider your choices and set some boundaries.

Personal Boundaries

Setting boundaries in your personal life related to your exercise and food choices can present many challenges. But personal boundaries communicate your needs in relationships, personal space, and express limitation.

These boundaries also include those you place on yourself to draw a defined line between behaviors that are constructive or destructive towards your habit alteration efforts.

Defining and limiting to what degree you are willing to expose yourself to instigators will be important in personal boundary setting. Special family gatherings and holidays are the most explicit and obvious examples where one should set some clear personal boundaries.

This is because gatherings with friends and family are usually strong instigators for indulgence and social pressure to eat or drink in a particular manner. Having set boundaries for yourself beforehand will help you make decisions with your intended outcome as a focus.

One boundary I set is not eating snack foods mindlessly at a party. I choose how much I will indulge and then I set a limit and stick to it. I prefer a good glass of red wine over cookies, candy, or chips, so that is how I set my boundary.

Of course, my whole family and group of friends know my profession and I rarely get ridiculed or pressured in those environments. This leads me to another boundary I set, which is disallowing people to excessively tease or ridicule me for my personal food choices.

As I mentioned in an earlier chapter, this happens quite frequently anytime I participate in fundraisers, events, mixers, or other social gatherings outside of my normal circles.

Once people find out I am a fitness professional, they scrutinize and even question every decision I make and what is on my plate. It's quite irritating.

Thankfully, my family and friends are not an issue anymore because I set those boundaries. I make the point because friends and family can be huge stumbling blocks for many people, and establishing that boundary is necessary. I hear stories from clients quite frequently about how hard it is to get family and friends to understand their boundaries and goals.

They get teased, pressured, or receive discouraging comments, which causes many to just cave in or create uncomfortable moments. There are quite a few ways you can go about setting and holding the line. Let's look at the two opposite approaches as an example, Silent Boundaries, and Formal Boundaries.

Silent Boundaries

First, we choose to covertly set limits internally and do not openly discuss or communicate boundaries through words. Instead, we set them by making better choices and allowing people to observe our behavior. They almost always do and may ask you about your decisions. It's painfully predictable, especially if you are making better choices than you have historically. People are curious or nosey and will likely ask you about it if they do notice.

This is a great method if you want to avoid conflict based on your family or friend dynamic. I like this approach as I should not have to explain myself or justify my personal choices related to wellness. I am not seeking to avoid conflict or discussion, as I will happily explain the basic benefits of my choices.

Yet, at a party or gathering, I do not want to debate diet theory, get made fun of, or have all my choices examined by people who can't even manage their exploding waistline or simply do not know what the hell they are talking about. This happens quite a bit with fitness and nutrition, where almost everyone believes they are an expert and pretend to know what you should or should not be eating.

Anyhow, actions speak louder than words, so my behavior is m preferred boundary communicator not what I tell people. The bonus to this is that only the observant will notice any of your choices, so you have less opportunity for interference from others. But on occasion, I must use a formal boundary to express the limit of my tolerance.

Formal Boundaries

The second approach to communicating boundaries is more formal, and I have seen this work for lots of folks. A formal way is where you have a family meeting or a direct conversation with a friend about your boundaries.

The upside to this is you can gain immediate and specific support from your sphere or expose areas for negotiation. The downside is that everyone now knows and will be watching because you formalized intent.

This may serve as a means of support or accountability and for that, there is a great value. Once, a client was struggling to create boundaries in her home and was getting little support from her husband and children.

She tried to be subtle and cleaned the house by removing all the junk foods and other instigators. She also scheduled her workouts and would complete them early in the morning so she could get her activity in and then focus on the day's events.

One of the biggest issues for her was dinnertime because she could not get her family to stop eating poorly and share in her healthy meals. She would prepare a chicken salad with dressing on the side for herself, but her family would order a pizza.

After the first week, junk foods appeared in the house again and because of her food choices, the family teased her by calling her a "rabbit." Adding to the frustration, her workouts got interrupted because the family noticed the pattern of her up and about in the morning, so they began to make other demands of her time.

She would start a workout and without fail, one of her children would interrupt and want to talk or make some other request. None of the children's needs were important at the time, and it was just a lack of courtesy because they did not recognize the silent boundaries.

By the third week, she had slipped back into eating pizza and was skipping workouts. Her boundary-setting approach was not strong enough to reduce instigators or gain support. Her habit of eating poorly and not exercising reemerged because she did not override the automation long enough to make real change.

In the fourth week, we were on a coaching call and strategizing how she could get back on track but also get her family to support her. We decided to go the formal path. She felt it best to tell her husband exactly what she was trying to accomplish and how he could help.

She wrote it out on a single piece of paper and had bullet points outlining her reasonable needs. Once she gained his support, they held a family meeting to discuss some of the changes they were going to make as a family and set clear boundaries.

Her children are adolescents and early teenagers, so they understood what she was expressing. They agreed as a family that pizza will only be once per week, and they will eliminate all soda and junk food from the house.

They came to a compromise on dinner because the kids did not like her food, but she made variations to accommodate everyone. They also agreed to make their lunches so she could get her workout in every morning. Which I forcefully suggested because why are you making your 14-year-old son a lunch? He can do that his damn self.

It was also clarified that she was not to be interrupted during her workouts unless it was an emergency. By week five, she was back to one hundred percent exercise adherence and her food intake was spot on. She now enjoys pizza about once a week, and they will sometimes swap pizza for another family indulgence.

It has now become something they look forward to and she has not experienced any major relapse since. Formal and clearly defined boundaries were perfect in her situation.

Boundaries for Pets

I can't believe I feel compelled to write this out, but it is a massive growing issue. The last note I will make on personal boundaries is regarding pets. Over the years, I have seen more people include the care of their pets as a priority of their wellness.

Folks, your pet is fine while you do a workout or spend extra time in the gym to develop your wellbeing. In fact, including pets in your outdoor activities is a great way to add more movement and improve their health as well.

However, it is not recommended that you prioritize a pet over yourself. You should set boundaries with your pets, just like you would with friends or family. I have had clients miss workouts, neglect their food management, and lose life focus because of a pet's demands. Ugh, this is becoming so common I had to write the last paragraph. Unbelievable.

Professional Boundaries

Strong professional boundaries are especially important because our careers can take up three-fourths of our day and present many opportunities for making poor wellness choices. You can use the silent, formal, or another effective approach based on your unique company culture.

Some of the common areas we should consider with professional boundaries include meeting snacks, lunches, dinners, cocktail mixers, and so on. Usually, this is just a personal boundary you must set internally and can be very transparent to your colleagues or clients.

In previous chapters, I review several methods for managing work-related outings where instigators or peer pressure may be present. Here I would like to simply remind you, you control what or how much you consume in meetings or work functions.

This section is really to cover something a little more complex, which is setting boundaries on your time, availability, and willing capacity in career expectations.

Work-life Balance

When I review exercise adherence with a client on a coaching call and I see missed workouts, they are nearly always related to their career. The circumstances are infinite and nearly every profession will experience some periods of long hours, additional workload, or looming deadlines. I can appreciate the occasional focus on work, putting in the time to complete projects and preserve a livelihood.

However, there should be strict boundaries placed around the duration or frequency of these intrusions. Sadly, many people sacrifice family, friends, and their wellness for a career. It is a tough mindset to overcome not to mention coaching people through.

I understand all the reasons and ways we can justify prioritizing our careers over just about anything, but I have never seen this bring joy. I encourage you to seek a balance between the trinity of life, which is yourself, your career, and your personal relationships.

Of course, within yourself, you can add spiritual balance, which should go without saying, but I want to be clear. Defining boundaries that support your total wellness and intended outcome in life will help you bring balance.

Without the vision of who you want to be and how that looks starts with boundaries. Take time to reflect on ways you can set boundaries aligned with your life plan. Balance follows boundaries.

Chapter Keynotes

Setting personal and professional boundaries allows you to communicate to others how you expect to be treated. However, you must create boundaries for yourself as well. Boundaries can be clearly expressed verbally or through your reactions to pushed or crossed lines. Boundaries also relate directly to your sense of self-worth and will be necessary for habit alteration.

- Internally, boundaries help us adhere to our values, physical and emotional wellbeing, and maintain our self-identity.
- Externally, boundaries help us communicate what is or is not acceptable behavior from others and help define our environments.
- Boundaries should not be set at the expense of excluding wellness; they should be seamlessly integrated into your lifestyle and translate to personal and professional dynamics.
- Defining and limiting to what degree you are willing to expose yourself to instigators will be important in personal boundary setting.
- Silent boundaries are when we choose to covertly set limits internally and do not openly discuss or communicate boundaries through words. Instead, we set them by making better choices and allowing people to observe our behavior.
- A formal boundary is where you have a family meeting or a direct conversation with a friend, colleague, or even your boss about your limits.
- You should set boundaries with your pets, just like you would with friends or family.
- Strong professional boundaries are especially important because our careers can take up three-fourths of our day and present many opportunities for making poor wellness choices.

- I understand all the reasons and ways we can justify prioritizing our careers over just about anything and neglect professional boundary setting, but I have never seen this bring joy.

PART II

Chapter Eleven
90-DAY HABIT
TRANSFORMATION WORKBOOK

This workbook assists you in developing a detailed plan to discover your primary motivators, address your readiness to change, and plan specifics to achieve your intended outcome related to habits.

You can break this out into weekly focus sessions or fill it out in one go. In my client coaching, I assign a portion as weekly homework so we can go through responses together and make each component manageable.

But if you are ready to get moving and have all the week one checklist done and ready, feel free to dive in. I have found when a client revisits their initial answers and goals after a period, their responses change as they grow.

I recommend going through this workbook several times each year to stay on point with your changing life.

Week One Action

Setting the Stage

In the first week, we will take some time to set the stage and get a system in place to maximize your effectiveness progressively. A common mistake many people make is taking on more than they can handle or process when they start a fitness or nutrition plan. In week one of this program, complete the following.

☐ Read Part I of **"The 90-Day Habit Transformation – The Essential Guide to Personal Improvement and Sustainable Wellbeing"** by Michael S. Parker.

☐ Reflect or write out some of the damaging internal conversations or comments you make to yourself that you would like to improve.

☐ Consider negative aspects of your external environment and how you will address reducing the negative effect of things mostly out of your direct control.

☐ Download and set up a nutrition and food tracking app or outline a journaling system.

☐ Have a professional write you a specialized meal plan or simply build your own and be prepared to execute this plan in week two. This plan should be calorically appropriate for your activity level and lifestyle. Be prepared to fully commit to your meal plan in week two and beyond.

☐ Choose one plan and shop for that single plan at first to reduce the risk of feeling overwhelmed and eliminate potential waste. I understand variety is important, but that comes later. For now, your goal is to stick to one plan for a short period until things start clicking.

☐ Have your exercise program written by a professional or ensure your workouts are appropriate for your condition and projected outcome. Workouts start at the latest in week two but may start in week one.

☐ Schedule your workouts and have a means of tracking your sets, reps, tempo, weight lifted, and exercise selection.

☐ Adjust your attitude to a positive and highly motivated mindset and be prepared to joyfully execute each week.

Week Two Action

Goal and Reward Setting

Setting goals and understanding your initial motivation towards them serves as a foundation for long-term success with the inclusion of discipline. There are many theories on human goal setting and motivation, and while they all have merit, I like to keep goal setting and motivation simple and personally applicable. For our purposes, I think of motivation and goals in two forms, the avoidance of pain and the pursuit of pleasure.

First, we are missing something or experience dissatisfaction, potential loss and are momentarily motivated to change our situation.

Second, we are momentarily motivated by outcomes, desires, or improvements to our lives. In both cases, we are seeking to optimize our well-being physically and mentally. Motives related to fitness and nutrition differ from a drive, so it's important not to mix them up.

A drive is deep and primal such as reacting to starvation, thirst, or injury, and so on while motivation is simply an emotion. We will look at motives that relate to more wellness-based mental or social outcomes and can be controlled deliberately through the Power of Conscious Response in our relatively comfortable modern lives.

Intrinsic Goals

Goals should be Intrinsic, which means the very nature of working towards a result in itself is a reward. The journey is just as, if not more important than the destination. These intrinsically motivating goals are exceptionally reliable when combined with discipline and provide more long-term fuel for achieving results. The motives come from within and are tied to personal mastery and purpose.

For example: working towards doing 10 pull-ups from zero provides a sense of accomplishment as even a single pull-up from zero is a reward. The excitement of slowly adding more pull-ups as you work towards your goal is intrinsically rewarding which causes the effort to be self-perpetuating.

Yet we must be aware that all motivation is temporary and fleeting so we must create as many opportunities as possible to recognize results by establishing milestones or being objective about progress toward a particular goal. Intrinsic motivators are a great catalyst for change and by their very nature, provide more frequent moments of success.

Extrinsic Goals

Extrinsic means the reward is the target result and working toward the goal is not a motive or necessarily enjoyable. Extrinsic goals can also be rooted in a desire to avoid a painful outcome, such as reducing the risk of disease. These motives are usually not strong and can wane quickly because the consequences are not immediate, and motivation is emotional. These motives are linked to outcomes such as reaping future rewards or avoiding potential pain.

For example: trying to lose 50 lbs in a specific time frame is a focus on the reward. Unfortunately, working off the excess weight is not enjoyable to you because of the manner of goal setting and realization of the time commitment it may take. The motive weakens under duration or by not meeting expectations for return.

While I rarely focus on external motives, we should address them so we can compare your internal motives because they may correlate, and one may give strength to another. You may also find that motives can shift, and it is important to acknowledge the potential change in a goal.

Refer to the chapter "Setting Realistic Expectations and Goals – The Motivation Myth" and "Developing Intended Outcomes" for guidance in this section.

In this section, outline at least three of your internally and externally motivated goals. Essentially, we must define not only the goal but why we have that goal. We must make these goals inclusive to ourselves and part of our conscious intention. In week three, we will dive deeper into goal intention and motivators.

Intrinsically Motivated Goal And Purpose	Extrinsically Motivated Goal And Purpose

Reward Structure

Now we must focus specifically on what actions you will consciously take to override your negative behavior or habit. This is where you will begin to apply some of the strategies found in The Power of Conscious Response. In this section, outline a positive reward structure that is sustainable and in line with your target outcome.

Almost anything can work as a reward if it fits into your budget and does not undermine your efforts. Food has been shown as a poor reward choice as it is often associated with instigators and a resulting negative habit, such as overeating.

Usually, food is so closely tied to an emotional cue that it can be counterproductive. I like to remind people we are not dogs, so think higher than treats. However, events such as a fancy dinner with a significant other to celebrate achieving a milestone can be a fantastic way to reward as the food is a secondary benefit to the experience.

Just be careful with it and make sure a special dinner date is aligned with your objective outcome. I use fancy dinners or restaurant experiences as a reward and form of celebration, and it works perfectly for me.

I never use single foods or snacks as rewards without it being tied to an experience. A reward should also be inspiring to you; otherwise, it will not compel you to stick to your plan. Here are just a few ideas:

A massage or spa day, new shoes, a new set of headphones, visit a friend, read a book, take a trip, indulge in a tech item, a concert, hire a housekeeper for a deep clean, hire a babysitter and go out or simply carve out a weekend or day for yourself. List at least three rewards you will give yourself for achieving milestone goals:

Rewards

Reward One	
Reward Two	
Reward Three	

Week Three Action

Six Fitness Cornerstones of Life

In this section, we explore the Six Fitness Cornerstones of Life which are linked directly to our motivation for achieving a goal. Once you outline your desires for each cornerstone, you will tie intrinsic motivators to each. This is a necessary part of goal setting. This discovery process is to uncover "why" you want to achieve a particular goal. Each motivator should end with "so I can..." or "because..."

Inclusivity is key to sustainability regarding your overall wellness, so these cornerstones serve you personally and professionally. Again, I recommend you do not focus on purely aesthetic outcomes or an arbitrary bodyweight number as a primary goal. The exception is if bodyweight is related directly to a potentially improved medical outcome.

One of the goals in this section is to understand your motivation and why you "feel" compelled to achieve a goal. Once you assess the motivation, sustainability or consistency will come in the form of developing Intelligent Discipline. Motivation is fickle, discipline can bridge the gap in goal milestones.

For some inspiration in this section, refer to the chapters "30x3+10 Rule" and "Wellness Consciousness" along with "Setting Realistic Expectations and Goals – The Motivation Myth" and "Setting Personal and Professional Boundaries."

Physical Fitness

The objective here is to maintain optimal physical health by remaining active and avoiding substances that harm your body. Motivators can be found here in athletics, physical skill, endurance, strength, flexibility, mobility, personal records, and potential longevity. This also includes the reduction or elimination of any substances that harm your body, such as narcotics, alcohol, or junk food. Below, outline three aspects of physical fitness that motivate you. (Example: I am motivated to do 10 full pull-ups because...)

Physical Fitness Motivator One	
Physical Fitness Motivator Two	
Physical Fitness Motivator Three	

Environmental Fitness

The objective here is to find ways of improving your external environment to align with your objective outcome. Motivators include adding to or building a home gym, lighting, workspace enchantment, or any other methods of encouraging adherence to your lifestyle goals.

This may also include the elimination of junk foods in the home or office, reduced television or social media usage and simply addressing any external instigators in your environments that may impede your progress. You may also find motivators in the addition or exploration of healthy food sources.

Outline three motivators related to your environment: (Example: I am motivated by eliminating chocolate from the house and office to reduce added sugar so I can...)

Environmental Fitness Motivator One	
Environmental Fitness Motivator Two	
Environmental Fitness Motivator Three	

Emotional Fitness

The objective here is to positively connect with your emotional responses so you can maximize them and create a disciplined strategy outside of those emotions. This includes how you see yourself, the content of internal conversations, how you deal with your feelings, and other forms of emotional self-love.

Motivator examples include improving your trustworthiness, attitude, confidence, perseverance, and eliminating negative self-talk. Outline three motivators related to your emotional fitness: (Example: I am motivated to stop calling myself fat or ugly when I look in a mirror because...)

Emotional Fitness Motivator One	
Emotional Fitness Motivator Two	
Emotional Fitness Motivator Three	

Spiritual Fitness

The objective here is to affirm positive beliefs, principles, humble virtues, or values aligned with your intended outcome as a human being. This can include adherence to religion, serving others, caring for animals, volunteering, or meditation. Outline three motivators related to your spiritual fitness. (Example: I am motivated to volunteer several hours to the local animal shelter because...)

Spiritual Fitness Motivator One	
Spiritual Fitness Motivator Two	
Spiritual Fitness Motivator Three	

Interpersonal Fitness

The objective here is to outline motivators related to the enhancement of romantic relationships, friendships, and familial ties. Some motivators here include communication, time, support, establishing boundaries, and compassion.

Finding ways to reciprocate and improve your sphere of influence starts with you. Outline three motivators related to your interpersonal fitness: (Example: I am motivated to include my partner in my desire to remain healthy by communicating my fears and new lifestyle goals because...)

Interpersonal Fitness Motivator One	
Interpersonal Fitness Motivator Two	
Interpersonal Fitness Motivator Three	

Intellectual Fitness

The objective here is to outline motivators related to the pursuit and application of knowledge, improve critical thinking, identify problems quickly and find solutions. This can include taking a course on a subject you are interested in, earning a certification, reading more books, researching, or generally engaging your cognitive abilities more frequently.

Outline three motivators related to your intellectual fitness. (Example: I am motivated to get an industry certification that improves my professional career so I can...)

Intellectual Fitness Motivator One	
Intellectual Fitness Motivator Two	
Intellectual Fitness Motivator Three	

Week Four Action

Instigator Discovery

Target behavior or habit change needs must be identified, and practical solutions should achieve your desired outcome. Sometimes, it helps to work backward by determining where you would like to be and then narrow down the root cause of habits impeding your life plan and desired personality.

For some inspiration in this section, refer to the chapters "The Power of Conscious Response" and "Wellness Consciousness" along with "Seven Intelligent Personality Traits."

Objective Negative Behavior or Habit Acknowledgment

Negative Behavior or Habit One	
Negative Behavior or Habit Two	
Negative Behavior or Habit Three	

Attainable Solution or Outcome

Positive Habit One Goal Outcome	
Positive Habit Two Goal Outcome	
Positive Habit Three Goal Outcome	

Next, identify and acknowledge cues (instigators) that start the cycle of each negative behavior or habit you wish to change. Recognize the internal and external instigators that initiate a subconscious or semi-subconscious set of responses.

The goal is to create new active reactions to these cues so you may practice overriding habits and replace them with outcomes aligned to your objective or desired future self.

First, we will examine your top three internally activated cues. This typically includes internal negative self-talk, results of decisions, attitudes, feelings, or opinions that may be hindering change or causing undesirable behaviors.

Internal Instigators

Internal Instigator One	
Internal Instigator Two	
Internal instigator Three	

Second, examine external instigators that elicit an undesirable response. These may include social situations, career, relationships, weather, living situation, finances, and other external factors largely out of your direct control.

External Instigators

External Instigator One	
External Instigator Two	
External instigator Three	

To drill down into more specifics related to your most recent internal or external instigator, use this simple journal outline for detailed discovery. Copy this questioning format to reveal details about future or past instigation.

Instigator Detail

Date, time, and location of instigation?	
Was it an Internal or External instigation?	
What are the details of the instigator?	
Persons Present during Instigation?	
What effect did persons present have on your instigation and response?	
What resulted from the instigation?	
How will you override the typical automated habit response in the future?	

Week Five Action

Solution Discovery

Now that you have outlined your top three internal and external cues, take time to reflect on the common situations and formulate a strategy to create deliberate responses to override your learned reactions.

In this section, you will write reasonable solutions or action items to combat these influencers so you can pro-actively work to replace your habitual response with a designed response attuned to your objective outcome.

For some inspiration in this section, refer to the chapters "The Power of Conscious Response" and "Developing Intended Outcomes" along with "Setting Realistic Expectations and Goals."

Internal Instigator One Solution	
Internal Instigator Two Solution	
Internal Instigator Three Solution	

External Instigator One Solution	
External Instigator Two Solution	
External Instigator Three Solution	

Remember, we must improve our internal environment before we can influence our external environment with some degree of control. In general, we must take personal responsibility for our actions and affect change there first. Once we have put our mindset into order, we are in a stronger position to affect relative improvement externally.

Do not get stuck in the trap of trying to fix or change your external factors first. It is a common mistake as we seek to avoid personal change and resist acknowledging our internal issues or faults. Not that we cannot formulate and execute a plan for improving external instigators, it is simply to remind you to focus on your internal shortcomings and prioritize accordingly.

Week Six Action

Are You Ready to Change?
The self-discovery of the first five weeks brings an intense level of awareness to your situation and place in your life vision. It may seem strange to have a preparedness evaluation in week six but the reason I usually identify this so late in the program is simple. Everyone thinks they are willing and ready to change until they see what it will take to make their goals a reality.

By assessing yourself and reconciling your goals, instigators, and the six cornerstones of fitness, you have arrived at the part that requires action which is the solution discovery in week five. Now that you know what it will take, are you ready to change?

For some inspiration in this section "Wellness Consciousness" and "Stages of Change."

True	False	
		1: I changed my Negative Behavior or Habit more than 6 months ago.
		2: I changed my Negative Behavior or Habit within the past 6 months.
		3: I intend to act in the next month and have made small changes already
		4: I intend to act against my Negative Behavior or Habit in the next 6 months.

Check below to see where you are in the Stages of Change for your listed Negative Behavior or Habits:

False for all four statements = **Precontemplation**
True for statement 4, false for statements 1–3 = **Contemplation**
True for statements 3 and 4, false for statements 1 and 2 = **Preparation**
True for statement 2, false for statement 1 = **Action**
True for statement 1 = **Maintenance**

What did you discover? Are you ready to put action on the discoveries you made about your habits and behavior so far? If you are ready to make improvements, move on to Week Seven and clean house. If you are not ready to act against your destructive habits, I encourage you to revisit your motivations, assess your goals and continue to Week Seven, and further your discovery. I hope you conclude through self-reflection to move forward in the Stages of Change. Don't give up!

Week Seven Action

Deep House Cleaning

Often, we must change our environments to suit our desired projected outcome. The classic saying of "Dress for the job you want" can be applied to your home and office environments related to fitness and nutrition. Discard the foods, drinks, or other negative instigators that can affect your ability to stay on point with your habit alteration. Shut off the television, power down the tablet, and get off your butt. Create environments for the lifestyle you want.

Case in point: I love chocolate and learned years ago that if it is in the house and available, I will eat it. I will eat all of it. The simple solution for me was to phase it out systematically and then not have it in my future environment. I went through an interesting and unexpectedly fun process to overcome my minor addiction to chocolate.

My mindset started to change after a candy-centered holiday where we had a significant number of leftovers in the house. So, I asked my significant other to hide it from me to keep it out of sight and mind.

But then she unexpectedly and on occasion, would put a little individually wrapped peanut butter chocolate cup next to my keyboard. I would sporadically find one on my nightstand or in my prepped lunch. Her creativity changed my association with chocolate and the game was incredibly supportive and thoughtful of her.

I valued the occasions she surprised me with the indulgence more than when it was just there and accessible. Something about the abstinence and unexpected appearance made the chocolate taste better somehow. I found out later she had discarded all the rest and only kept a few to share with me at random and I appreciated her support.

I then moved on to the second stage of habit alteration, which was permanently structuring my environment to support my efforts. Over a relatively short while, I overrode my cravings or desire for chocolate completely. Now, I never think of chocolate, nor do I get odd cravings that cause me to buy it. I have cleaned it from my house and removed any potential instigation or risk. Because of the consistency in which I apply this conscious response and how my relationship with chocolate changed, I can avoid eating it even when it ambushes.

I can now go to a party or event where chocolate is present and acknowledge it but abstain if I choose. Because I use the Power of Conscious Response in my life related to chocolate, I get to choose if I enjoy some and how much I consume. I have disconnected the unconscious response of consumption from this aspect of my life.

Oddly, I had a client once tell me she thought it was a weakness in character to need to clean house. She assumed that through sheer willpower, she could abstain from her indulgence in baked goods. I vehemently disagree with her for two reasons.

First, the very nature of consciously controlling your responses and environment by eliminating risk is precisely how we alter behavior. It's not a weakness of character to create boundaries for yourself; it is Intelligent Self-Awareness.

Second, if she possessed that willpower, then she would not have consumed a whole pan of brownies by herself in one sitting with a pint of ice cream, nor weigh in at near 260 lbs with 48% body fat.

Let's be objective and remember discipline and willpower are skills. In this section, write what items you will throw out and what items you will not bring into your environment.

For some inspiration in this section, refer to the chapters "Developing Intended Outcomes" along with "Setting Realistic Expectations and Goals."

List of Items to Remove from Environment

Items to Eliminate in the Future

Week Eight Action

Singular Habit Assessment

Truly consider your most destructive negative behavior or habit. Mark on the left side how it has affected you today and on the right column, outline how it will affect you in the future if you were to not make a change. In the second row, outline what the effect will be with instant change and what that change may look like over a period.

For some inspiration in this section, refer to the chapters "The Basics of Habit" and "Wellness Consciousness" along with "Setting Personal and Professional Boundaries."

Negative Affect Today	Negative Effect Long term
Positive Affect Today	Positive Effect Long term

Explore and deeply consider your resistance and mental defenses to avoid improvement. Resistances include denying the consequences of your negative behavior or habit and rationalizing your reasons for not changing.

Fear-based resistances can be a form of disruption in routine, fear of failure, fear of guilt, and fear of exhaustion. Reference the Part I chapter on Habit and Resistances for inspiration. List the mental habit resistance mechanisms you use to resist change:

Defense Mechanisms

Identifying a support structure is wildly helpful. Consider what family or friends have conveyed to you about your condition, habit, or behavior. List their names, who they are or mean to you, and what they said to you about your negative behavior or habit:

Name	What They Mean to Me	Things They Have Said About My Behavior

Examine your support structure or negative influences together. Are some of your family and friends a negative influence or detractor? You should lovingly communicate to those impeding your progress through their negative word or deed.

In extreme cases, you may need to create a degree of separation. Identify individuals in your sphere of influence you want to gain better support from on the left. On the right, list those you may need to disconnect yourself from or change the nature of your relationship with to achieve your positive habit outcome:

Positive Supporters	Possible Detractors

Many humans thrive on community support. List some local support groups or activities that can help with positive outcomes. This includes churches, topic-related support groups, leagues, or clubs of folks likely to support your efforts and provide positive reinforcement. List the groups you would like to be part of.

Defense Mechanisms

Week Nine Action

Visual Cues and Tracking

In this section, we will work to contemplate unique ways of exposing habits we wish to change through visual cues. Food or behavior journaling is a great way to visualize and map habits to illuminate the scope of your negative action and create an objective view.

There are quite a few technologies you can leverage to make journaling or data collecting quite simple. Apps for your mobile device and wearable tech all make it simple to get a good picture and help you understand your patterns.

At Forge, we use this data to look at food consistency, workout adherence and find patterns in the data. I can often look at a client's food journal and tell where they went off track very quickly so I can adjust coaching content accordingly.

This also allows for you to recollect what instigator caused the negative habit to manifest. If technology is not your thing, try placing all the wrappers or containers of junk foods you ate into a pile for a month and see how that affects you.

One client collected her wine corks in a large glass jar on her counter for a month so she and her family could see them. After it overflowed in less than a month, she was motivated to change her habit, so she consciously prepared to make a change.

List some strategies for visual contemplation you think would work for you below.

For some inspiration in this section, refer to the chapters "Developing Intended Outcomes" along with "Setting Realistic Expectations and Goals."

Strategies for Visual Contemplation

Cost and Value Assessment

Sometimes, evaluating the cost of your behavior or habit can be a gateway to the preparation phase. My clients are often surprised by the cost impact of their decision-making after stepping back and evaluating. But comparing cost is only part of the benefit of this exercise as you get to assess the perceived total value of your behavior as well. As an example, one of my clients had a daily coffee addiction. She would stop at a popular coffee shop at least once each day.

The average cost of her 600-calorie coffee was $4.75. Some days, she would have it twice, but for the simple math, we will examine the monthly cost in calories and money for 30 days. 600 calories x 30 = 18,000 empty calories monthly divided by 3,500 calories equates to over 5 pounds of potential body fat. This is if her total caloric intake were in surplus, but it's an alarming illustration. Now we look at the financial impact. $4.75 x 30 days = $142.50 given to a daily habit over a month. In a macrocycle of one year, she is consuming over 216,000 empty calories and spending around $1,710 on coffee.

After she completed the Pros and Cos, she decided the sum consequences were not valuable enough to continue the behavior. It took time, but she redirected her habit in phases and worked to cut off one day each week.

She replaced it with a far less expensive and dramatically lower calorie option at home, so she still had coffee each day. The problem was not coffee, it was the total calories and cost that was the damaging behavior in her assessment.

As a solution, she purchased a home coffee maker for $90 and a coffee pod that cost around 60¢ each day plus a splash of almond milk. Her daily coffee calorie intake went from 600 calories to approximately 45 calories. Let's look at the year, including the coffee maker investment. Her total calories for the year went from 216,000 to 16,200 and her cost went from $1,710 to $310.25 for the first year, including the coffeemaker. Complete the cost-benefit analysis worksheet:

Identify Monthly Monetary Cost of Negative Behavior or Habit

Pros of Negative Behavior or Habit	Cons of Negative Behavior or Habit

Pros of Making Change	Cons of Making Change

Now that we have a financial figure association and a benefits analysis, we can hypothetically redirect our financial resources positively. If the sum of your costly negative behavior or habit is eliminated, what would you do with the money normally directed towards your habit?

Financial Redirection

As a regular practice, we should strive to refine our self-image. Creating a positive and high-quality personality projection is a powerful way of envisioning who you want to become. In this exercise, describe the kind of person you will be in the first section and how your life will improve because of this change in the second.

Projected Self-Description	
Life Quality Description	

Now that you have contemplated the Pros and Cons of your negative behavior or habit, you can decide if you are prepared to improve. It may take some time in the contemplation phase, but don't give up! Keep working through your mindset and even if you must emotionally claw your way, keep moving toward change.

Week Ten Action

Strategy Review

Take some time to specify your plan with additional detail discovered over the past ten weeks. Be flexible to the concept of altering your plan as you progress. I find fluid plans are more effective than rigid because your goals may change as you discover more about yourself and project your desired outcome.

Take a moment to conceptualize your plan and put the framework in writing.

For some inspiration in this section, refer to the chapters "Developing Intended Outcomes" along with "Setting Realistic Expectations and Goals."

Specific Plan for Improvement

List of supporters who know of your plan. This includes family, friends, or hired professionals.

Name	Relationship	Role in Your Plan

Now that you have a plan to attack your objective with passion, sign, and date it. If you are so inclined, have a friend or your coach sign it with you. I know it seems silly, but it is a fantastic way to formalize your decision and a good step towards the concept of Intelligent Trust.

Week Eleven Action

Plan Adherence Accountability

Action is fundamental to all endeavors and plans without action are useless. In this section, outline how you will measure and manage your daily actions toward behavior change.

This can be food journals, workout logs, wearable technology data compared to food logs, body fat and lean muscle scans, or manual circumference measurements.

For some inspiration in this section, refer to the chapters "Developing Intended Outcomes" and "Setting Personal and Professional Boundaries" along with "Setting Realistic Expectations and Goals."

How Will You Track Progress?

How Often Will You Track?

Who Will You Share This Data With?

Reward Revisions

As we progress, you may find new ideas for rewards related to habit alteration. Reflect on the past ten weeks and revise any possible reward opportunities.

Reward One	
Reward Two	
Reward Three	

Week Twelve Action

Stress Management Strategy

Understanding your reactions to internally manifested or externally instigated stress will be a critical aspect of your total wellbeing. Stress causes cortical inhibition and affects cognitive quality, heart rate, pulmonary function, immune system, metabolism, digestive system, libido, and musculature.

Identifying stressors and consciously working to relieve that stress as quickly as possible is a skill that takes practice and awareness. I like to break stress sources into three categories so I can objectively prioritize action to combat stress.

Internally Manifested Stress

The stressors you have the most control over are ones you manufacture internally. This includes needless worry, doubt, fear, lack of sleep and even spending too much time on social media or watching toxic mainstream news.

Social media is a danger as it presents vast potential stress-inducing reactions. These stressors can be political, social, or economic. If social media routinely causes you to become angry, frustrated, offended, or provokes any other negative emotion, it's time to shut it down.

Career Related Stress

These include any aspect of your professional life, such as total work hours, commute time, professional relationships, job stability, income, the danger level of vocation, and so on.

Personal Relationship Stress

These stressors include finances, family, health, romance, living situation, logistics, and so on.

In this section, list your primary stressor and then a possible solution to that stress. I highly encourage you to think big and even if the solution seems insurmountable or difficult, it may be a sign you need to make a life change. For example, you may find that a solution is to end a relationship, change jobs or make significant alterations to your life. Do not fear creating a strategy as you must make these acknowledgments.

For some inspiration in this section, refer to the chapters "The Power of Conscious Response" and "Setting Personal and Professional Boundaries."

Stress Category

Internally manifested stress	
Career Relate stress	
Personal Relationship Stress	

Stress Solution

Internally manifested stress	
Career Relate stress Solution	
Personal Relationship Stress	

Week Forever

Maintenance

Maintenance is the stage in which people have successfully altered behavior and the action has produced results and they are working to prevent relapse. While in the Maintenance stage, people are less tempted to relapse and grow increasingly more confident they can sustain their new behavior and habits.

In addition, many people see a new manifestation of goals from elevated or improved lifestyles such as new athletic endeavors, outdoor activities, or other life-enhancing enterprises.

You must continue to monitor behavior in some objective fashion. Journaling is a great way to keep a record and compare trends related to instigators. Environmental management and keeping a clean house will go a long way to support you.

Most importantly, keep a conscious and deliberate set of responses to your known triggers while looking at every instigation as an opportunity. I welcome instigators because it allows me to practice my behavior or habit alteration and maintain resolution in acquisition and response.

Congratulations on completing this workbook and roadmap to sustainable fitness and nutrition success!

PART III

Chapter Twelve
WHERE TO START WITH NUTRITION

Proper nutrition is the foundation of a healthy lifestyle and critical to personal performance. Individuals must ensure their food intake is aligned with their lifestyle and personal goals by consuming whole foods with high nutrient density. This means avoiding fast foods, processed or pre-packaged-high preservative foods.

If you sacrifice quality for convenience, the results will show poor performance and declined health. Plus, many of these food sources serve as instigators for many people and can interfere with your habit alteration efforts.

I highly encourage my clients to choose foods such as vegetables, fruits, whole grains, lean proteins, and clean fats and take the time to prepare and plan meals.

Nutrition is so complex and a source of fad and contention, I felt it important to communicate the objectives of this chapter:

1- Explain in simple detail, exactly what macronutrients are and what they do in the body.
2- Explain how to estimate your calorie needs and expenditure, or Basal Metabolic Rate (BMR) and Total Daily Energy Expenditure (TDEE).
3- Expose some myths, the complexity, and misconceptions about nutrition.
4- Provide basic and well-known scientific information to support healthy consumption.
5- Outline each macronutrient simply and provide some basic examples of food sources so you are positioned to make better choices.
6- Common sense and education will empower you to make better nutritional choices and improve your relationship with food, so you understand how to make better

decisions regarding your food intake and avoid the fad diet trap.

Because this book was never intended as a scientific manual, scholarly article, or textbook, I have simplified the references by using the following textbooks instead of referencing every point throughout paragraphs in the book:

Nutritional References
- Caudill, M.A., & Stipanuk, M.H. (2013). Biochemical, Physiological, and Molecular Aspects of Human Nutrition: Third Edition, St. Louis, MO: Elsevier Inc.
- Smith, A.M., & Wardlaw, G.M. (2011). Contemporary Nutrition: Eighth Edition, New York, NY: McGraw Hill.
- Geissler, C., & Powers, H. J. (2017). Human nutrition. Oxford: Oxford University Press.
- Sienkiewicz, F & Whitney, E (2011). Nutrition Concepts and Controversies: Twelfth Edition. Sizer-Whitney.

Aside from the scientific references consolidated here. I would like to acknowledge Anna Bartholemy, RD, LN, CPT. She assisted with referencing, helped me organize content, and validate the chapters on Carbohydrates, Proteins, and Fats. She also kept me from over-explaining and keeping my word count reasonable. Thanks, Anna!

How to Choose and Estimate Caloric Intake Targets
First, estimate your Basal Metabolic Rate (BMR), or in some circles, Resting Metabolic Rate (RMR) is a great place to start. Your BMR is an estimate of your body's energy needs to maintain primary functions such as breathing, circulation, cell production, and nutrient processing. Essentially, it is a close guess calculation to determine what you may expect your body to burn at full rest.

Once we identify an approximate BMR, we can apply an estimated Total Daily Energy Expenditure (TDEE). This will help you determine your likely caloric output based on your activity level and exercise structure.

The common approach for calculating BMR is with the Harris-Benedict formula, which considers weight, height, age, and gender. You can also use the Mifflin-St Jeor equation if you prefer but I did not include that here. I provide the constants in the equation for both Imperial and Metric so just fill in the variables and complete the arithmetic.

Imperial Equation
Women: BMR = 655 + (4.35 x weight in pounds) + (4.7 x height in inches) - (4.7 x age in years) = BMR of: _____

Men: BMR = 66 + (6.23 x weight in pounds) + (12.7 x height in inches) - (6.8 x age in years) = BMR of: _____

Metric Equation
Women: BMR = 655 + (9.6 x weight in kg) + (1.8 x height in cm) - (4.7 x age in years) = BMR of: _____

Men: BMR = 66 + (13.7 x weight in kg) + (5 x height in cm) - (6.8 x age in years) = BMR of: _____

Total Daily Energy Expenditure
Now we add an energy output multiplier to estimate our potential calorie expenditure each day.

Sedentary: You get minimal or no exercise, multiply your BMR by 1.2.
Lightly active: You exercise lightly one to three days a week, multiply your BMR by 1.375.
Moderately active: You exercise moderately three to five days a week, multiply your BMR by 1.55.

Highly active: You exercise vigorously six to seven days a week, multiply your BMR by 1.725.

Extremely active: You exercise extremely hard six to seven days a week and/or have a physical job, multiply your BMR by 1.9.

Now that you have a basic understanding of your potential calorie output, choose a meal plan that satisfies your daily need compared to your desired outcome. See the various meal plan examples in the "Additional Resources" chapter of this book.

Basic Nutrition Concept for Fat Reduction

If your goal is fat reduction, it is advised you maintain a deficit of 250-650 calories each day. This complies with the basic Laws of Conversion of Mass, wherein your body has achieved a certain output of energy that exceeds intake.

Because the energy was used, your body must make up the deficit to balance the energy equation to neutral. In this case, it is hopefully the conversion of stored energy or fat that will make up that deficit.

As a note of caution, less is not better. A common mistake many people make is cutting too many calories and creating an excessive deficit. This is shown to lower your metabolic rate and cause fat retention, not fat loss.

Conversely, too much energy intake and you have a surplus. The body will store this excess as fat. Energy is not created or destroyed, it simply alters its nature like water to steam and back again.

Basic Nutrition Concept for Muscle Development

Unlike fat reduction, the development or hypertrophy of lean muscle tissue requires energy as you are building the body and need material to do so. Naturally, this material is in the form of nutritional components and energy. Everyone is a bit different, but it is generally ideal to at minimum, meet your maintenance energy or exceed it slightly.

Maintenance energy is simply the equality of calories consumed compared to calories expended. You will need to ensure you have a sufficient and balanced ratio of carbohydrates, proteins, and fats to ensure maximal absorption and distribution of nutritional building components.

It is indeed possible for many people to reduce body fat while simultaneously adding lean muscle tissue. It requires some diligence and keen observation of your biofeedback, but it can be done. Be sure that your intake is not excessive as this will add body fat if in consistent surplus. Your training paradigm must include structured resistance training to maximize this outcome.

How to Read a Nutrition Label

Understanding the basics of a nutrition label will empower you to make informed decisions about your food choices. There are four key areas to observe on the label including serving size, calories, nutrition, and daily values.

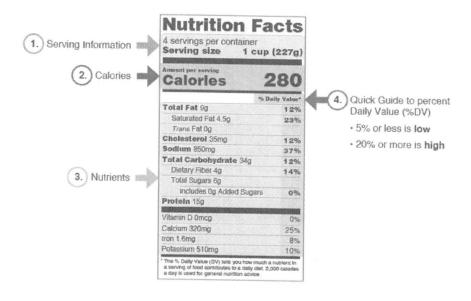

Serving Information

First, we want to identify the serving size of the product. Serving sizes are displayed in common measurements such as cups followed by a metric measurement such as grams. The serving size is not a recommendation for how much one should consume, but an estimation of how much one might typically consume.

It is especially important to pay attention to how many servings there are in the package, otherwise, you may accidentally overconsume. For example, if you are about to consume a product that displays one serving as 3 ounces, but you consume 6 ounces, you would need to double the nutrient and calorie amounts, as well as the percent of daily values, to calculate your intake. This is a common oversight so keep an eye on the servings per container.

Calories

The number of calories is the total amount of energy the food provides. Each macronutrient contains several calories per gram. Carbohydrates and protein contain 4 calories per gram and fat contains 9 calories per gram. A high-calorie food does not necessarily mean it is bad for you. However, one should limit high-calorie foods rich in saturated fats, trans fats, and added sugars. As a side note, Alcohol contains 7 calories per gram.

Nutrients

Americans typically eat too much saturated fat, trans fat, refined carbohydrates, and sodium, which can increase the risk for heart disease, cancer, or diabetes. Use the information provided on nutrition labels to help you choose foods containing less than 10% of calories from saturated fat and added sugars.

You should aim to get more fiber, vitamin A, vitamin C, calcium, and iron in your diet. Strive to consume 15-20 grams of protein at each meal, this is especially important if you are exercising.

These nutrients may reduce the risk of developing chronic disease and help manage body composition. It is recommended to consume 100% of each of these nutrients daily to prevent nutrition-related diseases.

Percent of Daily Value

Understanding the Percent Daily Values (% DV) on a food label can help you choose foods high in optimal nutrients and low in more undesirable nutrients. The % DV is based on a 2,000-calorie diet. If you eat less than 2,000 calories a day, your daily value may be lower than what is listed on the label.

If you eat more than 2,000 calories a day, your daily value may be higher. 5% DV or less is low and 20% or more is high. Choose foods with a low % DV for fat, saturated fat, trans fat, added sugars, cholesterol, or sodium. Choose foods above 20% DV for vitamin D, calcium, vitamin A, iron, and fiber.

Carbohydrates: The Truth

To start, we need to explore what carbohydrates are and how they affect the body from a cellular standpoint. Understanding the intricacies of carbs will allow you to make more informed decisions about carbs in your dietary lifestyle.

Carbohydrates have been the relentless target of the modern media scorn and have been improperly classified. The demonization of carbohydrates is simply the product of ignorance, gullibility, and greed, which leads to consumer exploitation.

Carbohydrates have been grossly generalized and lumped into a singular group without delineation for monosaccharide, disaccharide, and polysaccharide or food source quality.

In addition, popular media and many fitness products or services ignore microbiology and manufactured fad diets that appeal to fear or a desire to justify consuming outrageous quantities of bacon as an alternative.

Before we get into the details, let us just dispel some myths right away. This is not a comprehensive list, just some of the top myths I run into:

Myth: Carbohydrates Are Bad for My Health

Carbohydrates make up the most nutritious foods on our planet. Yes, carbs predominate cookies, candies, and baked goods, but they are also the major macronutrient in fruit, vegetables, and whole grains. Carbs are our only source of dietary fibers.

Dietary fibers help us maintain normal gut function protect our heart and helps us manage appetite. It is the processed carbs (added sugar, cake, cookies, refined grains) that when overeaten lead to chronic disease. One should aim to get 45-60% of their calories from carbs for optimal health.

Myth: Carbohydrates Make You Gain Weight

Carbohydrates cause your body to release insulin, which puts you in an anabolic state, meaning your body stores energy. This insulin response is critical to optimal cellular function and energy production. Without it, you would feel fatigued, and sugar may be retained in your bloodstream, possibly causing hypertension and kidney damage.

Often people lose weight when they cut out carbs because they deplete their glycogen stores. Glycogen is the storage form of carbohydrates in muscle and liver, but it is mostly water. You are losing the 3-4 pounds of water bound in your glucose storage when you suddenly cut out carbohydrates, not necessarily body fat.

Myth: I Should Avoid Gluten

Gluten is in wheat, barley, and rye. It is a protein contained in carb-rich foods. Recent research has shown gluten may or may not have an autoimmune response. Gluten-free diets are often recommended to persons with irritable bowel syndrome, polycystic ovarian syndrome, Hashimoto's disease, and celiac disease.

A growing number of people have gluten sensitivity, but if you do not experience bloating, abdominal pain, or brain fog after eating gluten, then there is no reason to cut this food out of your diet.

Myth: Bread and Pasta Must Be Eliminated

Refined grains of bread and pasta do not need to be fully eliminated. They should, however, be portion-controlled. A portion of bread equates to one slice and 1/2 cup is a standard portion for grain. This portion contains approximately 15 grams of carbohydrates.

Eating a slice of bread occasionally will not make or break your nutrition plan. Many dietitians recommend one should aim for 40-60 grams of carbohydrate at each meal to maintain proper blood sugar levels.

Myth: All Carbs Are Created Equal

Depending upon the fiber content, carbohydrates break down to sugar at a slow or fast pace. If there is no fiber, such as a cookie, then your blood sugar will spike and drop rapidly. This will cause you to feel hungry again quite soon. If you are choosing whole grains such as whole-wheat bread, brown rice, quinoa, bulgur, starchy vegetables, and fruits, then fiber will slow down digestion.

Your blood sugar will rise over a few hours keeping you feeling satisfied longer while also supplying you with necessary vitamins and minerals.

Carbohydrate Structures

Now that some of the big myths are cleared up, let's dive into some of the simple sciences related to carbohydrates. Not all carbohydrates are created equal, and one objective is to share with you the difference between complex carbohydrates, which comprise sugars, starches, and fiber versus those made of simple carbohydrates which contain one or two simple sugars.

Despite the complexity, all carbohydrates contain 4 calories per gram. At the core, carbs are compounds composed of single or multiple sugars chemically shortened to CHO signifying carbon, hydrogen, and oxygen.

The configuration of each carb will determine its complexity, digestibility, and glycemic yield. Complex carbohydrates meet your body's energy needs, feed your brain, nervous system, and keep your digestive system fit. Within calorie limits, they help keep your body lean because carbs are also protein sparing.

Meaning carbs protect against excessive gluconeogenesis, which is the function of converting non-glucose-based components into glucose, such as your muscle. Carbs also help reduce nitrogen in the system, such as urea, which burdens the liver and kidneys in excess. Carbs also aid in cellular respiration by facilitating, with insulin, the transport of molecular energies through the Citric Acid Cycle and the production of adenosine triphosphate, or ATP through the Electron Transport Chain.

ATP is an organic chemical that provides energy to the cell. However, the Citric Acid Cycle and Electron Transport Chain are so complex it was by far the most challenging biological function for students to grasp when I was teaching college and I will not be diving any further into those topics in this book.

So, let's talk complex versus simple carbs. The very basic sugar unit is a molecule containing six carbon atoms together with oxygen and hydrogen to make monosaccharides and bonded pairs that makeup disaccharides. Complex carbohydrates have long chains of sugar arranged to form starch or fiber. These are called polysaccharides.

Essentially there are six common sugars in nutrition. Three of which come from monosaccharides, and the other three come from disaccharides. There are other sugars such as xylose, ribose, and so on, but we will keep this basic. You have likely heard many common sugar types as they all end with "ose" which essentially means sugar.

While sugar types may sound similar, they each exhibit very distinct characteristics. Glucose is the most popular and well-known name for sugar followed by fructose, galactose, lactose, maltose, and sucrose and those are the carb sources we will explore here.

Glucose is a single sugar used in both plant and animal tissues for energy. Fructose is commonly called fruit sugar. Galactose and Lactose are milk sugars. Maltose is known as malt sugar. And finally, sucrose, also known as a table or cane sugar.

And that, my friends, is the sugar, along with high fructose derivatives that are highly addictive and the source of the "carbs are bad" nonsense. I acknowledge there are a fraction of people with a sensitivity to carbs, are medically pre-dispositioned, or do not feel their best with a higher carb diet. Everyone is different so find what works.

Simple Carbohydrates

Popular simple carbs include the raw form of products containing: Sugar, brown sugar, corn syrup, and high-fructose corn syrup, honey, glucose, fructose, and sucrose, and that nasty fruit juice concentrate.

Mono sugars can be found in refined quantities in mainstream food sources such as soft drinks, cereals, baked goods, enriched white bread and pasta, candies along with hundreds of other products. Even your spaghetti sauce is loaded with sugar.

Let's break it down even further with some basic chemistry as it relates to each of the sugar types so we can have a better understanding of why some forms of carbohydrates are preferable to others.

This will expose how and why we experience carb confusion. The common monosaccharides include glucose, fructose, and galactose. The molecular arrangements result in degrees of sweetness, with fructose being the sweetest.

I should point out that the total volume of fructose in fruit is not significant enough for most people to exclude or even minimize fruit in their diet. This is related to the glycemic load and insulin response, which we will cover shortly and debunk the myth "fruit is bad because it has sugar."

Yet, if you are inactive and overeat, even fruit can contribute to excess energy that leads to fat accumulation. Usually, the fruit did not cause fat gain, it was perhaps the half-gallon of ice cream underneath the fruit or the six ounces of chocolate sauce. Not the fruit.

Complex Carbohydrates

Now let's do a quick overview of Disaccharides, which include lactose, sucrose, and maltose. Another interesting distinction between monosaccharides and disaccharides is how they are absorbed by the body.

Monosaccharides are absorbed directly into the bloodstream, so you get a big blood sugar spike, while disaccharides must go through a period of digestion first, they still boost blood glucose levels high but just a tad less than a monosaccharide.

We have intestinal enzymes that split the bonded pairs into separate monosaccharides so they can enter the blood. Next, they make their way to the liver, where they are converted to glucose then are used or stored. In lactose, glucose is linked to galactose.

Malt sugar or maltose has two glucose units. Finally, there is sucrose, commonly called table sugar. In sucrose, fructose and glucose are bonded together in a refining process typically from Juices, sugar beets, or sugarcane, and appear in small quantities naturally in several varieties of fruits and vegetables.

But it's the manufacturing process that bonds the fructose to the glucose making for super sweetness and hyper addiction. It's very important to point out that while we derive energy from sugar in fruits and many vegetables, this does not mean eating them is the same as consuming concentrated sweets in soda, candy, and other forms of highly refined sugars.

There are other forces at work here, including starch, fiber, and hormonal response to food type. It's also important to recognize the total volume of glucose response from watermelon compared to soda is vastly different even though they share identical glycemic indexing.

But before we get into the insulin response to glucose ingestion and glycemic index and load, we need to cover complex carbs, starch, and fiber because they play a critical role. Complex carbohydrates contain a longer series of sugars that the body takes longer to break down.

That means you will release lower amounts of sugar into your bloodstream at a more consistent rate. Foods with complex carbohydrates typically contain greater values of vitamins, minerals, fiber, and starch.

You must be careful because these crafty food manufacturers sneak stuff into packaged foods. Check nutrition labels for no added sugars, enrichment, or fortification. I know enrichment and fortification sound positive, but they are not as they are part of processing and destroy nutritional density in foods. Not to mention genetically modified foods.

Popular whole food complex carbs from tubers and grains include oatmeal, yams, and sweet potatoes, brown rice, multigrain, potatoes, 100% whole wheat bread and pasta, beans and lentils, quinoa, and couscous.

On the fruit side of the complex, we have examples such as grapefruit, apples, blueberries, cantaloupe, oranges, bananas, peaches, grapes, strawberries, pineapple, blackberries, pears, and so on.

Popular complex veggies include broccoli, kale, asparagus, spinach, peppers, onions, mushrooms, cucumbers, zucchini, carrots, and cauliflower. These are all excellent sources of complex and nutritionally dense carbs with great fiber and starch.

Starch

Starch is simply a plant polysaccharide composed of glucose. After some denaturing (cooking) starch is highly digestible and critical for digestive health. Starch is essentially a plant-stored form of glucose, and as a plant matures, it provides energy for itself and seeds. Starchy foods are a great source of energy and a prime source of nutrition in our diet.

Plus, starches contain fiber and a whole host of micro-nutrients. Many starchy foods such as potatoes, bread, rice, pasta, and cereal have been falsely classified by pop culture as fatty.

The reality is gram-for-gram starches contain far fewer calories than any fat source, fat = 9 and carbs = 4 calories per gram. This is another great example and misconception about carbohydrates and their relationship to over-fatness or obesity crisis.

I concede, it is quite easy to consume significant quantities of carbohydrates in a day so serving size plays a critical role. It's important to remember that starch-based carbohydrates are first converted into glucose, then glycogen, or if you over-consume, it will be stored as body fat. Law of conservation of mass.

This is where portion control and an active lifestyle can be extremely helpful by utilizing that glucose and assist in caloric energy balance or deficit depending on your fitness or composition goals.

A final point on starch: there is another type of starch called "resistant starch" with four classifications and they include Type 1: in grains, seeds, and legumes.
Type 2: in raw or unripe food sources.
Type 3: cooked then cooled rice or potatoes that become more resistant because of retrogradation.
Type 4: which are artificially manufactured through a chemical process.

Fiber

Like starch, nearly all fibers are polysaccharides just chains of sugars, but they're different from starch because the sugar units are held together by bonds the human digestive enzyme cannot break.

But billions of bacteria in the large intestine do possess enzymes that can digest fiber to some degree through fermentation.

Here are some examples of some very high fiber foods: barley, oatmeal, oat bran, seeded fruits like apple, banana, blackberries, nectarine, orange, peach, pear, plum beans like black beans, kidney beans, navy beans, and our lovely veggies such as broccoli, brussels sprouts, carrots, asparagus and so on— all affordable and accessible.

Fibers are broken into two groups based on their chemical, physical, and functional attributes. The first group of fibers we will discuss are soluble, so they dissolve in water. Through dissolving, they form a viscous gel, which can be digested by bacteria in the colon through fermentation.

On the other end, we also have Insoluble fiber, which does not dissolve in water, so it doesn't create that viscous gel because of resistance to fermentation. Insoluble fibers are in the outer layer of whole grains, stringy vegetables, seeds, and plant skins.

These insoluble fibers even retain the rough texture after cooking and aid the body with digestion. The point is fiber-rich foods provide significant benefits. Whole-grain foods, vegetables, legumes, and fruits deliver valuable vitamins, minerals, and phytochemicals plus digestive benefits.

Fiber is attributed to the promotion of normal blood cholesterol, control of blood pressure, thus reducing the risk of hypertension, modulation of blood glucose concentrations, maintenance of healthy bowel functions, and the promotion of healthy body composition.

The Glycemic Factor

The glycemic index (or GI) is a ranking of carbohydrates on a scale from 0 to 100 according to the degree they raise blood sugar levels after eating.

Foods with a high GI are those which are rapidly digested and result in spiked blood glucose levels like monosaccharides or disaccharides. Low GI carbohydrates produce smaller fluctuations in your blood glucose and insulin level, like polysaccharides.

Now, you have the glycemic load of food, which is a number that estimates how much the food will raise a person's blood glucose level after eating. Think of it as an intensity gauge. One unit of glycemic load approximates the effect of consuming one gram of glucose. GL is based on the glycemic index and is calculated by multiplying the grams of available carbohydrate in the food multiplied by the food's GI and then dividing by 100. Here is a mathematical example:

Watermelon has a GI of 72. A serving of watermelon (154g) has 11g of available carbohydrates making the calculation: 11(g) × 72(gi) / 100 = 7.92 grams of available carbohydrates (calories = 46)

Cola has the same GI of 72. A serving of Cola (368g – 12oz) has 39.8 available carbohydrates making the calculation: 39.8(g) × 72(gi) / 100 = 28.6 grams of available carbohydrates (calories = 140)

One year I had a student point out the serving disparity of 154 vs 368g in my nutrition class. Even if you matched gram for gram serving, you still only increase the GL of watermelon into the moderate range at approximately 16 and it still doesn't break 100 calories. 368g of watermelon would be 2 ½ cups.

I will also point out; most folks don't eat 2 cups of watermelon but can slam a couple of twelve-ounce cans of soda with a total caloric intake of 280 and a glycemic load of 57.2.

This expresses that while some fruit may share the same glycemic index as a portion of junk food, the hormonal and glucose responses are quite different.

Let's talk hormones. Once carbs are absorbed into the bloodstream, you also release insulin. The rise and fall of blood glucose and the duration it remains elevated is the glycemic response. Complex carbs and minimally processed starchy foods produce a different response than the simple carbs, as we just discovered with the watermelon and soda example.

Other factors include how much food you eat in a sitting, how processed is the food, and even how the food is prepared. But insulin and glucagon work together to create metabolic homeostasis.

If you get a huge spike in sugar, you get a huge spike in insulin. The moment your insulin is released, you are no longer converting stored energy. This includes body fat. Glucagon is released as glucose levels drop and bring the body back to homeostasis.

I want to express how incredibly I am over-simplifying this but understanding the basics will help you put this all together. So, the height and frequency of your elevated blood sugar will directly correlate to your ability to convert body fat for energy, technically named lipolysis.

The Nutrition Facts Label also lists the types of carbohydrates that make up the total carbohydrate in a product. This includes the dietary fiber and sugars and the percent of the daily value.

Some labels include soluble and or insoluble fiber, sugar alcohols, and "other carbohydrates." which are usually starch. Here are some Food and Drug Administration (FDA) guidelines: The Daily Value for total carbohydrates is 300 g per day. This is based on a 2,000-calorie diet and may not be the right serving size for you.

The goal is to get 100% of the Daily Value for total carbohydrates but your daily value, not a generic average. The FDA points out: 5% DV or less of total carbohydrate per serving is low and 20% DV or more of total carbohydrate per serving is high.

But do you need 300g of carbs? I don't. I typically look for 200g for myself, so about 800 calories of my intake can come from carbs on a sedentary day, and I will bump it up if I am very active or on a backpacking trip.

Also, there is some research showing that most humans have a better cognitive function with 130g or more of carb intake. You can do a web search on that and see some peer-reviewed articles with interesting findings.

And if you didn't know, carbs are broken down by total grams per serving and the percent of Daily Value on a nutrition label so pay attention to that and most importantly, total sugar as those will be simple sugars.

In conclusion, carbohydrates are not good or bad, but some are much better than others. However, your decision-making related to food type and volume of consumption can be good or bad. I remind folks they must take personal responsibility for their fitness and nutrition.

Carbs don't make us fat; our choices make us fat. I understand so many people are struggling with body fat and composition management, and I empathize. Even I go through periods of challenge and frustration.

For most of us, it used to be a lack of information, but now with the media and the internet, there is more misinformation than fact. As a culture, we seek the easy path and when our consumption turns on us, we keep the same "I want it now" mentality and look for shortcuts, fad diets, excessive food source exclusion, pills, or gimmicks that promise immediate success. It's all false and taking advantage of your vulnerability and pain. If you want to stop that pain, you own it.

And if you have a medical condition that carbs aggravate, then keep tuning your food intake until you find the right combination. Get active for at least 150 minutes each week and do not eat more than you expend and make better choices related to carbohydrates and all food types. It takes time to do it right and permanently.

Protein: The Truth

Protein is in every living cell in the body. Our bodies need protein from the foods we eat to build and maintain bones, muscles, and skin. We get proteins in our diet from meat, dairy products, nuts, and certain grains and beans. Get enough dietary protein, especially if you are active and performing weight-bearing exercises. Before we get into the details, let's expose some myths related to protein.

Myth: I Am Not Getting Enough Protein Throughout the Day

Most people get enough protein throughout the day but may not consume protein frequently enough. There is no storage form of protein in your body, and we can only absorb 20-30 grams of protein at once.

That is why it is so important to eat protein frequently throughout the day. One should aim to have 20-30 grams of protein 4-5 times a day or 1 gram of protein for every kilogram of body weight.

Dispersing your protein intake throughout the day will lead to maximum benefits in the maintenance of muscle, satiety, and neurotransmitter production.

Myth: Protein Powder Is the Best Route for Muscle Building

Your body utilizes proteins more effectively from whole foods, which also supports the intake of vitamins and minerals. It is often recommended that individuals working to gain muscle should drink protein shakes if they do not have another option, or if they are having trouble consuming the necessary calories for hypertrophy. But shakes and bars are simply supplementing and should not be your primary protein source.

Myth: Too Much Protein Causes Kidney Disease

Protein, unlike carbohydrates and fats, contains nitrogen. Nitrogen is quite acidic, and our kidney brings blood back to the baseline by excreting nitrogen from protein as ammonium found in urine.

This process does not damage our kidneys unless one were to consistently intake three times their daily recommendation. It would take significant effort and overindulging in protein to have negative consequences.

Myth: You Can't Have Too Much Protein

Protein is an important macronutrient, but it cannot directly replace carbohydrates and fat. Protein is a great source of minerals but often lacks water-soluble vitamins and fat-soluble vitamins. Protein consumption is also tied to animal products, so there are some large ethical questions or personal preferences one may consider.

While eating lean meat and dairy is a great source of protein, many people already over-consume these foods due to misguided portion sizes. For example, 3 oz of meat contains 20-25 grams of protein. 3 oz of meat is about the size of a stack of cards. While it is important to get protein-rich food at each meal, more protein does not equal more or faster results.

Myth: Protein Is the Best Post-Exercise Meal

Protein should be included in one's post-exercise meal, but the body uses glucose to fuel workouts. We want to also replenish our carb storage to maximize the efficiency and assimilation of proteins. Eating a combination of carbs and protein is the best recovery meal.

Many vegans and vegetarians often struggle with options for recovery meals, but there are several plant-based sources of protein include soybeans, lentils, tofu, quinoa, oatmeal, barley, pea protein powder, seeds, fish, eggs, tempeh, hemp, and Greek yogurt. Vegan or not, these can be combined and prepared beforehand for quick whole food snacks without using animal products or supplements.

Protein Structures

Proteins like other macromolecules comprise of carbon, oxygen, hydrogen, and contain a nitrogen molecule. Amino acids are the building blocks of protein, they bind together via peptide bonds, which defines their function.

The sequence of these amino acids will determine how a protein will fold. The fold of a protein, or structure, determines its function. Our bodies produce eleven amino acids on their own, and there are nine essential amino acids we must consume from food, twenty in total.

It's possible the foods we had access to historically are what made essential amino acids, essential. The foods we ate determined the functions of our bodies over time. Amino acids were one of the first organic chemicals on this planet, along with nucleotides, the components that makeup DNA/RNA.

These molecules are linked to almost every process that makes a living organism alive. Nucleotides make our DNA, and DNA made it possible for our bodies to combine amino acids into structures called protein.

The process that started it all is called transcription. In transcription, our DNA creates RNA. This can occur because DNA molecules are in the structure of a double helix or spiral. It comprises identical sequences of nucleotides. When the body needs protein, our DNA, which holds the recipes for every type of protein in the human body, unwinds.

RNA copies the needed strand of DNA (directions) verbatim. It mimics the exact sequence of nucleotides except it replaces the T nucleotide with a U. This allows the RNA strand to communicate with amino acids. The copied RNA strand is ready to be used in translation.

The mRNA is taken out of the nucleus and into the cytoplasm where it binds with a ribosome, which can then translate the RNA into a protein by sequencing amino acids. The sequence of the amino acids determines how the protein will fold and the fold of the protein defines the function.

Whenever our bodies need an enzyme, a blood cell, or an antibody, this process occurs. This process is not perfect and sometimes malfunctions in protein synthesis occur at no fault of our own. For example, we can think about the translation process, which converts that message of the RNA sequence and determines the folds of the protein.

If the protein has an amino acid misplaced, it will change the structure of the protein. This would cause a misfolded protein that is unfunctional. With brain cell function, these misfolded proteins can no longer properly function and form plaques within the brain, which can be a cause of degenerative diseases such as Alzheimer's. On the other side of the coin is a malfunction in protein synthesis caused by diet. If we are malnourished or deficient in essential amino acids, we can see some of these issues arise.

However, not eating enough protein in a single day will not cause any of these problems. These symptoms of malnutrition only occur when we do not eat enough protein for months or when we have an illness that increases our protein needs. Yet, we should always aim to meet our minimum protein needs to help our body function at the optimal level.

Daily Recommendations

The standard recommendation for protein is 0.8 to 1.2g per kilogram of body weight. Each body is unique and different, having its own needs that should be considered. For those that are not highly active, and the body is not taxed or under distress, the 0.8 recommendation may be adequate. For children, highly active adults, athletes, the elderly, those interested in losing weight, instances of malnutrition, we can see clients thrive at a higher than the recommended 0.8 per kilogram intake.

For many athletes, protein needs may be closer to 1.0-1.7 grams per kilogram. Unfortunately, it cannot be as clear and black and white, because of the complexity of the unique nature of the human body. Recent evidence has shown that our bodies can only absorb 20-30 grams of protein at once even if we are an athlete or sedentary individual. This occurs because protein is very acidic in our blood due to the nitrogen molecule. Our bodies will excrete nitrogen in the form of ammonium to protect the pH of our blood.

The best way to ensure you are maximizing protein absorption is to eat protein at each meal. For example, if you weigh 80 kgs and are trying to consume 1 g of protein per kilogram of bodyweight, then you should eat 20 grams of protein 4 X a day. Or 25-30 grams of protein at each meal. This will also ensure that your body is in control of its blood sugars and regularly creating important neurotransmitters, such as serotonin.

However, if you are not a performance athlete or working on highly specialized food intake for a specific goal, it is unnecessary to be so precise. Simply spread your protein intake out and shoot for a reasonable total percentage or grams each day. We should eat intuitively and in a balanced manner without crossing the line from conscious discipline into needless obsession over finite details.

Too much or too little

If you often feel tired, constantly hungry with cravings between meals, then you may not be getting enough protein. Protein can be a negative factor if you consume far too little for extended periods or far too much. If our protein intake is consistently inadequate, we may experience physical signs such as weak and brittle nails, hair loss, white spots on the nails, low blood pressure, fatigue, cognitive lapses, immune deficiencies, and depression.

On the other hand, if you feel heavy, bloated, and sluggish after meals, then you may be getting too much protein. If we have an extreme intake of protein daily, we may experience renal failure because of the increased workload on the kidneys, which filter waste products from protein metabolism. Gout or uric acid build can be a sign of too much protein in the diet with an increased buildup of waste products from amino acids with higher concentrations of purines.

High amounts of protein in the diet can also cause increased acidity in the body with calcium excretion. But again, these factors are only for extreme and consistent protein deficiencies or overconsumption. But these are extreme examples, and you are unlikely to experience the effects of protein deficiencies or surplus.

Amino Profiles

Dietary proteins can be split into two categories, complete proteins, and complementary proteins. Complete proteins will contain all the essential amino acids. Our complementary proteins are those that need to be combined with other forms of protein to get all the amino acids needed.

All animal products are complete proteins so when consuming this protein source, you will not have to worry about getting the variety to meet your amino acid needs.

There are several vegetarian sources of complete proteins as well, such as quinoa, potatoes, soy, and wheat germ. Complementary proteins do not contain all the essential amino acids and come from vegetarian sources such as beans, legumes, nuts, seeds, grains, and peas. You will have to eat a variety of these proteins for them to be complete and have all the needed amino acids.

Complementary Proteins include lentils, almonds, cabbage, oats, chickpeas, sesame seeds, spinach, whole wheat, peanuts, sunflower seeds, cauliflower, corn, peas, cashews, avocado, barley, beans, walnuts, brussels sprouts, and rye.

As a side note, there is a debate in the dietetics community regarding the validity of complementary proteins and amino profiles. Because not all the research on this topic is conclusive and people smarter than I am are studying it, I will wait to amend the standard teaching protocol until there is definitive proof.

Vegan/ Vegetarian

One tip for our plant-based friends is the need for variety. When considering complementary proteins, we should look at our complete dietary consumption to ensure maximal nutrient intake. If we are eating a reasonable variety of plant-based proteins, our amino acid pool will be adequately fueled. It is a myth that vegans and vegetarians do not get enough protein for skeletal muscle development. This is especially true with the advent of dozens of options for vegan-friendly protein supplementation.

Protein Supplements

I am personally not a fan, but I also do not necessarily discourage the use of protein supplements. Utilizing a quality protein supplement may be useful to those who train and want to maximize their muscular development, as well as for individuals lacking protein in their diet.

Remember that protein supplements do not contain the naturally present vitamin and minerals in whole foods, and we don't know if the labels are accurate or truthful. In my opinion, whole-food sources are always best, but protein shakes are a convenient tool for supplementing your diet.

When choosing a protein supplement, consider the digestibility of the protein, allergens, processing, protein quality, and ingredient lists. Regarding whey, you may see things like hydrolyzed, isolated, concentrated, or grass-fed.

Whey Isolate protein will be filtered so only pure protein and the amino acids remain but not as concentrated with the other molecules in whey. Due to the manufacturing process, it is more highly refined and contains greater amounts of protein. Hydrolyzed whey protein has been shown to aid in absorption time and digestion. Grass-fed and organic can be important to those that are interested in keeping their diet clean of pesticides and other potential additives.

Since toxins are stored in the fats of animals, it might be worthwhile to choose an organic whey or one that is isolated so there are fewer chances of remaining fats in the protein source.

When thinking about a vegetarian protein supplement, I typically recommend an organic form, if not, there is a high probability you are drinking up all those pesticides used on the farm along with your protein.

Soy is a protein that is revered by some for the alleged healthy benefits associated with your heart and hated by others for its estrogen properties.

If consumed daily, it is always beneficial to make sure it is not Genetically Modified Organisms and organic when possible. If you are concerned about hormonal disruption, monitor your hormone levels to ensure it isn't having estrogenic effects.

Pea protein is favored by many because it is affordable and abundant. If you are having digestive issues such as IBS or bacterial imbalances, pea-based protein may be problematic for some. Hemp has the benefits of Omega 3 fatty acids, and rice proteins can be easily digested.

The bottom line with all the types of vegetarian proteins, it's important to be diligent about reading labels and make sure it has the nutrient quantities you're looking for to find the best fit for you.

Protein powders often contain excessive additives and fillers, so I recommend checking the label of your protein source.

Read labels carefully for things like gums, natural flavorings, lecithin, colorings, and so on. Identify your favorite type of sweetener whether it is stevia, monk fruit, coconut sugar, and so on.

Also, look at the sugar count on the label as well as any artificial sweeteners such as dextrose, sucralose, saccharin, and so forth. Some people may be particularly sensitive to sugar alcohols such as xylitol and erythritol, so pay attention to your body's response. All in all, the more simplistic the ingredients list, the healthier it probably is, but it is a food supplement, not whole food, so you get what you get.

Fat: The Truth

At one point in time, the concept of incorporating butter and oils into our cooking for better health would have made people run for the hills. The truth is quality fats have always been a major part of a balanced diet. Fats create our hormones which are responsible for the signaling and communications among our cells, and they allow us to absorb vital nutrients necessary for our health. In this section, you will learn why fat is so important to our bodies, what is considered high-quality fat, and the foods in which to find them.

History

Once upon a time, fats were deemed bad for our health. For many individuals who grew up in the 1970s, their childhood was marked by the taste of skim milk, margarine, and egg whites. In 1977, the Senate committee passed its landmark "Dietary Goals for the United States." The number one recommendation was to avoid cholesterol and fats of all kinds. The directive was backed by a 150-million-dollar study that linked fat consumption to heart disease.

In reaction, grocery stores stocked low-fat dairy products, eggs were replaced with breakfast cereals, and carbs became the new staple in the American diet. These changes did not help to reduce the risk of heart disease.

Chronic disease became more prevalent during this time with type II diabetes almost tripling in the United States. Intuitively the idea that consuming fat makes you fat would make sense. Compared to other macronutrients, fat is most dense in calories.

While carbohydrates and proteins have 4 calories per gram, fat has 9 calories per gram. For many dieters and individuals that grew up during the war against fat, the paradigm that fats are bad for you is deeply ingrained in our psyches. As is the concept that eating fewer calories causes more weight loss, which is untrue. Science has caught up with nutrition and human metabolism and has confirmed fat is an essential part of our diet.

Before we dive deep into the science of fat metabolism and composition, let's explore the unconscious and conscious beliefs you may have instilled in your mind regarding fats. Do you unknowingly choose reduced-fat products? Do you choose margarine over real butter? Do you lean toward whole eggs or egg whites? Do you opt-out of seeds and nuts in oatmeal to reduce calories? What causes you to make these food choices has less to do with conscious decision making, and likely more to do with the conditioning of our society in mainstream diet culture. Let's set it straight and dispel these common misconceptions about fat.

Myth: Fat Is Not Needed in The Body

Like every other macronutrient, fat is essential in our diets. Fats have an integral role in hormone functions, gut health, immune response, reproduction, nutrient absorption, and cell communication.

Myth: Dietary Cholesterol Raises Cholesterol

Food sources high in dietary cholesterol do not have a positive correlation with raising cholesterol. High cholesterol occurs when people consume diets high in trans fats and sugars because they interfere with the body's natural ability to recycle cholesterol. Cholesterol is used to create estrogen, testosterone, vitamin D, and create important immunity proteins and are essential for health.

Myth: Eating Dietary Fat Increases Weight

This idea could not be further from the truth. Research shows that people who eat moderate amounts lose just as much if not more weight than people on low-fat diets. This occurs because fat allows for slower digestion and decreased insulin release, especially when paired with a higher glycemic food.

Myth: Eating Fat Will Increase Risk of Heart Disease

Excessive intake of trans fats and sugar will lead to an elevated risk of heart disease; natural dietary fats that are unsaturated reduce one's risk of developing heart disease by reducing bad cholesterol called Low-Density Lipo Proteins (LDL).

Myth: More Fat Consumption Is Better for My Health

On the other hand of the fat myth, ketogenic diets have become very popularized and high-fat diets have increased. Ketogenic diets are indicated for certain disease states and may be recommended by a dietitian or medical practitioner. Ketogenesis is achieved when glycogen stores are drained, and you are eating less than 25 grams of carbs a day in which your body is fueled by ketone bodies.

This diet is not recommended for most people because it is hard to get the necessary nutrients and may be unsustainable. There is such a thing as too much fat, so unless your doctor has prescribed a ketogenic diet, aim for 20-35% calories from fat.

Fat Structures

Similar to carbohydrates, much of the confusion with fat lies in the numerous types. There are saturated, unsaturated, triglycerides, short-chain fatty acids, long-chain fatty acids, and so on. Let's simplify this for this book. 95% of dietary fats in our food intake are in the form of triglycerides.

A triglyceride consists of a glycerol backbone and three fatty acids. Fatty acids come in many different forms. There are three main categories: unsaturated fatty acids, saturated fatty acids, and trans fatty acids.

Saturated fats

These fat types are predominantly from animal products and can also be found in coconut oil. A good way to pinpoint saturated fats is that they are solid at room temperature. There is a lot of mixed research regarding saturated fats. Once, saturated fat was believed to be the single culprit behind high LDL levels or "bad cholesterol." Yet, recent research has indicated this is not entirely true.

Moderate amounts of saturated fats are okay in the diet, specifically from sources such as coconut oil, full-fat milk, and butter. The dietary guidelines recommend that less than 10% of your calories come from saturated fats.

Unsaturated fats

Predominantly from fish and plant fats, these sources are well known for having positive health benefits. Unlike saturated fats, unsaturated fats contain a double bond in the structure. The number of double bonds in the structure dictates if the fat is monounsaturated, which contains one double bond, or polyunsaturated, which contains multiple double bonds. Monounsaturated fatty acids are well known to reduce the number of LDL in the bloodstream and increase levels of "good cholesterol" called High-Density Lipo Proteins (HDL).

Food high in monounsaturated fatty acids includes olive oil, eggs, avocados, nuts, and seeds. Polyunsaturated fatty acids can hold several different double bonds. The most important polyunsaturated fats are omega 3s, which contain three double bonds. Food high in omega 3 polyunsaturated fats includes fish, seafood, seeds such as flax, soybeans, and sunflower.

Trans fatty acids

Not found naturally in most foods, small amounts can sometimes be found in dairy, but they are mostly manufactured in a process called hydrogenation. Manufacturers favor hydrogenation to stop oxidation of oils from occurring which increases the product shelf-life. These hydrogenated oils are also resistant to breakdown in hot temperatures giving food products like fries a particularly crispy texture. Trans fats are most common in fast food and processed foods such as cookies, cakes, doughnuts, and chips.

These are unhealthy types of fats because of their negative effect on the body, lack of nutritional quality, addictive properties, and added empty calories. Trans fats have been banned in most European countries because our bodies cannot process these manufactured fats.

If time and heat cannot break down these chemicals, our body most likely will not either. Consuming trans fats is associated with tissue inflammation, insulin resistance, weight gain, digestive issues, and it raises LDL cholesterol and lowers HDL. The American Heart Association advises limiting trans fats to less than 1% of calories. I recommend even less.

Most of the fat we consume is compiled in a molecule called triglyceride. The triglyceride has a combination of fatty acids. Unsaturated fatty acids are the most beneficial to your health, saturated fatty acids are okay in moderate amounts, and trans fatty acids are correlated with disease.

Specifically, heart disease. So why might early scientists have correlated natural fats to disease and weight gain? Trans fats were almost nonexistent in our food supply during this time. To understand the emerging research on fats, one must first understand how fats are digested in the human body.

The triglyceride enters our body, travels down the esophagus into our stomach where it is primed for digestion. The fat molecule moves into the small intestine where our pancreas releases an enzyme called lipase. This enzyme breaks apart triglycerides into their building blocks of fatty acids, glycerol, and cholesterol.

The fatty acids attach to fat-soluble vitamins such as A, D, E, or K which carry them along for absorption. These vitamins could not be absorbed without the presence of fat. Our body then comprises these building blocks into a chylomicron, which can travel freely through the body. The chylomicron moves into our bloodstream and travels to organs and muscles that need immediate energy. If we eat in excess, they will be stored as fat for use as energy later just the same as carbohydrates and protein.

There is nothing specifically that causes dietary fat to be stored at a higher level than any other macronutrient. After chylomicrons supply our bodies with immediate energy, they will return to our liver. What is left inside the chylomicron are cholesterol, fatty acids, and vitamins. The liver uses these compounds in both HDL and LDL.

They deliver nutrients, cholesterol, and fatty acids to different cells in our bodies. These compounds are needed to create prostaglandins or sex hormones, immune compounds, and lipids to build the cells in our brain. Another fun fact about fat is that our brain is 60% fat and assists with integral cell communication and signaling.

HDLs or the "good cholesterol" comprised of protein and some cholesterol. They move through your blood and pick up extra cholesterol in your circulatory system. They move this cholesterol to useful places like back to your liver and to your pancreas to help you create bile acids or prostaglandins.

LDLs or "bad cholesterol" are directly associated with heart disease, obesity, and high-fat diets. Yes, the consumption of fat increases LDL levels, but scientists have recently discovered there are two different types of LDL cholesterol. One type of LDL is large and fluffy, the other one is small, dense, and sticky.

The large fluffy LDL has been deemed harmless to our health in recent years. The small LDLs are the lipoprotein most associated with adverse health risks. They are dense particles composed mostly of cholesterol molecules. They have a strong affinity for depositing in our arteries, building plaque-causing atherosclerosis and hypertension.

So, what causes your body to produce this small toxic LDL versus the benign LDL? Trans fats have been found as the culprit here. Trans fats not only increase toxic LDL but also decreases the production of HDL. The second cause is when we have a diet high in added sugar. Added sugar increases insulin release and insulin causes our bodies to shift into storage mode. Namely, storage of cholesterol into floating LDL also while increasing serum triglycerides.

Some research has shown that saturated fats can cause a deficiency in the binding mechanism to LDL. This causes LDL to continue to circulate, unable to attach to cells and deliver nutrients. So much for low-fat diets preventing heart disease! The discovery of the two different types of LDL cholesterol turned this 1980s myth on its head.

Daily Recommendations

The dietary guidelines recommend 20-35% of your calories come from fat. There are three general guidelines to help aid you in meeting this goal with quality fats. First, consume 3 servings of fat at each meal aiming for 8-12 total servings a day. A serving of fat is a tablespoon and there are 5 grams of fat and 45 calories in a serving.

Second, incorporate mostly unsaturated fats into your diet, which include fish, flaxseeds, avocado, olive oil, sunflower oil, safflower oil, walnuts, almonds, and pistachios. Third, eat saturated fats from sources such as eggs, butter, coconut oil, and full-fat dairy products and aim to have less than 10% of your total calories from saturated fat sources.

Finally, eliminate trans fats! Read labels. These can be hiding in peanut butter, microwavable foods, and even popcorn. Implementing these guidelines into your lifestyle may feel daunting and are simply to provide a blueprint to optimal nutrition. True changes happen by awareness and incorporation of small changes one at a time. A great first step would be to build awareness around your fat intake and the type of fats you are eating by reading food labels to better understand what is in the foods you consume.

Omega 3 supplementation

Many Americans get enough omega 6 fatty acids in their diet but neglect and to get enough omega 3s. Omega 3s can be found in salmon, walnuts, flaxseed, chia seeds, and seafood and most Americans do not get enough. If you do not eat 2-3 servings of fatty fish a week or at least a tablespoon of flaxseed a day, you are most likely deficient. In clinical settings, supplementation is indicated when persons have signs of heart disease, depression, and hormone imbalance, such as high estrogen or low testosterone.

If you experience any of these disease states, your body is already deficient in this key nutrient. Omega 3 intakes may help prevent the onset of Alzheimer's, joint inflammation, and plaque build-up in the arteries. Some dietitians recommend everyone take an omega 3 supplement if they are in a deficiency.

When choosing a supplement, you are aiming to meet the need of 1 g -1.5 gram of EPA combined with DHA a day. EPA and DHA are more active forms of omega 3. You can take a fish oil capsule, flaxseed oil, ground flaxseed, or aim to meet your weekly fish recommendations of 2+ servings a week.

Hydration

The American Council on Exercise has suggested the following basic guidelines for drinking water before, during, and after exercise:

• Drink 17 to 20 ounces of water 2 to 3 hours before you exercise
• Drink 8 ounces of water 20 to 30 minutes before you exercise or during your warm-up
• Drink 7 to 10 ounces of water every 10 to 20 minutes during exercise
• Drink 8 ounces of water no later than 30 minutes after you exercise

Clients may want to measure how much fluid they lose while training to get a more specific measurement of how much water to drink - 16 to 24 ounces of water for every pound of body weight lost.

Signs of Dehydration

Dehydration results from expelling more water than you consume. When your body doesn't have enough water, it can't work properly. Dehydration can range from mild to severe with symptoms ranging from:

- Dizziness or lightheaded feeling
- Nausea or vomiting
- Muscle cramps
- Dry mouth
- Lack of sweating
- Hard, fast heartbeat

Symptoms of severe dehydration can include mental confusion, weakness, and loss of consciousness. Also, darker-colored urine may be a sign of dehydration.

MICHAEL S. PARKER

Chapter Thirteen
PRACTICAL NUTRITION CONCEPTS

Our bodies are very efficient machines that exist by converting the energy and properties of other organisms and then adding the nutritional values of carbohydrates, proteins, fats, fibers, vitamins, and minerals to our cells. Because of this direct conversion, we are what we eat.

The quality of food, nutritional density, and caloric value of food sources all play a role in healthy nutrition. The availability of food in American culture and the method in which it is prepared to play a significant role in the prevalent increase in obesity. In addition, many people are unaware of or simply ignore the quality or calorie content of the foods they choose.

Fast food, saturated fats, processed and preserved foods along with sugars and sodium-filled foods are easily accessible and well branded. The attraction and instant gratification in many of these food items can be hard to resist or eliminate from one's diet. Here are 5 Simple Steps to get on the path to healthy eating:

Commit to Yourself and the Plan

The first step on the path to healthy eating is to deeply commit yourself to the duration, menu, and structure of a clean eating program. Often, our dietary habits are formed over long periods and are very much a part of our daily activities and unconscious behaviors. We can come up with a handful of creative excuses on why we don't or feel we can't, commit to better food choices.

We often blame schedules, children, spouses, convenience, finances, or even lack of nutrition knowledge. These excuses are not extraordinarily strong, and you can work to overcome excuses and prioritize your wellbeing. It's a hard truth, but once the commitment is made to improve one's nutritional intake, it becomes much easier to focus on the following steps to improve lifestyle and wellbeing.

Clean House

Once the commitment is made to healthy eating, the first action must be purging your home of any foodstuff not fresh, wholesome, or otherwise high in calories and low in nutritional value. Some of the obvious offenders include highly processed foods such as frozen pre-packaged meals, snack cakes, chips, cookies, ice creams, granolas, candies, sugar drinks, and any of the myriad of other culprits lurking in your kitchen.

Food high in sugar, sodium, or calories must be eliminated, and if you take the time to read nutrition labels and be honest with yourself about the quality of foods in your home, it may be staggering to uncover the low quality and high-calorie foods you have collected and consumed. Often, people seeking body fat loss or improved nutritional intake see a degree of success by simply banishing poor quality foods and making better meal choices at home.

Choose Nutrition Over Calories

Now that you have made the commitment and cleared away the temptations and pitfalls of low-quality foods in the home, you can assemble a high nutrient and low-calorie menu plan.

Optimal nutrition requires a balance between carbohydrates, proteins, and fats where these macronutrients can be obtained through lower-calorie options. Some complex carbohydrates with high nutrient density and low calories include barley, quinoa, whole grains, chickpeas, yams, beans, and vegetables.

A few excellent complete proteins include eggs, skinless chicken breast, lean turkey, salmon, cod, tuna, buffalo, pork tenderloin, and combining complementary sources such as black beans and brown rice for a vegetarian protein option. Excellent fats include avocado, pecans, walnuts, almond butter, and oils such as coconut, olive, and flaxseed.

There are many variations and countless other options for quality carbs, proteins, and fats listed above, so do some homework and find the high-nutrient, low-calorie food sources that best suit your tastes and ability to prepare.

Pre-Plan & Time Balanced Meals

Now that you have the best ingredients, it's time to plan your meals for each week and be sure to get a good balance of all the main macronutrients. The 2010 Dietary Guidelines for Americans recommends eating within these ranges: Carbohydrates: 45-65% of calories, Protein: 10-35% of calories, and Fat: 20-35% of calories. It is critical to balance the proper number of calories consumed to the ideal ratio of macronutrients.

One's resting metabolic rate, activity level, and wellness objective should be tied closely to nutritional intake. The best way to ensure consistency and keeping on track is by planning and preparing meals in advance. Meals should be prepared on a Sunday for the following Monday, Tuesday, and Wednesday. Thursday, Friday, and weekend meals should be planned or prepared by Wednesday evening.

As for timing, it is often best to eat at regular intervals of three to four hours to ensure a maximal supply of nutrition and energy delivering calories. Without question, water must be added to this consideration and regularly consumed to feed the body process and brain function.

Add Variety and Keep It Fresh

There is much debate over the subject of dietary variety in academic circles. Some argue variety keeps the body from under-processing common food sources based on efficiency adaptations while some contend that altering one's normal routine can adversely affect digestive microbes.

And the list of arguments and debate grows with the mounting glamorized demonization of glutens, fats, carbohydrates, or other popularized food villains. Regardless, humans have a remarkable ability to consume a wide range of foods and sometimes variety just keeps eating from becoming monotonous.

Spicing it up makes it much easier to stay on the clean and lean path. Provided you keep within your caloric range, proper macronutrient ratio, and do not suffer from a pre-existing condition, variety should not be a challenge.

Chapter Fourteen
WHERE TO START WITH FITNESS

Weight Training Fundamentals

With over 52.9 million Americans working out in a health club, less than 13% work with a certified fitness professional, and 44% who quit working out annually claim it is related to lack of results because they "don't know what to do" or an injury they acquired while exercising (IHRSA, 2014). It was this statistic, among others, which caused me to conceptualize Forge. I knew there had to be a way to make personal training more accessible or affordable for the thousands of people who try and fail to achieve their fitness needs.

Anyway, one of the biggest mistakes made by nearly all gym-goers is applying the incorrect weight training strategy as it relates to their goal. Usually, people turn to the internet, magazines, or friends for workout advice. This is possibly the worst way to start a program as these resources often suggest a program outside the condition of the questioning individual or are scientifically unsound.

Unfortunately, the average American is significantly deconditioned, and most popular programs or fad workouts are overly intense and inappropriate because the "Acute Variable" is incorrect for that person.

The 6 Levels of Fitness Hierarchy

The human body is a complex machine capable of remarkable performance and generally responds in a very predictable manner. On one hand, if we are sedentary and consume more energy than we use, we can expect to store body fat and experience system deconditioning. On the other hand, if we apply the right acute variables in a specific manner, we can predict physiological outcomes.

From a practical safety standpoint, deconditioned individuals with poor mobility, flexibility, and stabilization will likely suffer from a series of dysfunctional moment patterns and possess lower integrity through the range of motion, thus increasing the chances of injury. Plus, you never want to layer strength over dysfunctional movement.

A common mistake many people make when starting an exercise program is the incorrect application of acute variables related to their condition and goal. If your goal is to be an Olympic weightlifter, then it will not be appropriate to work out like a basketball player. Your outcome will be very disappointing, but the good news is, it's all quite predictable.

Likewise, if you have been sedentary for some time and decided to start a workout program, be careful to select the acute variables in the program design that take your current condition into account while preparing you for more advanced movements and loads.

To help with this concept, let's look at the Fitness Hierarchy of program design. I use this approach daily in my fitness and nutrition practice as it reduces the risk of client injury and maximizes the efficacy of their efforts with predictability.

Mobility

Biomechanical mobility is the ability of a joint to move optimally through the proper range of motion without restriction or altered reciprocal inhibition from surrounding tissues. Joint function or arthrokinematics are foundational to advanced flexibility, stability, and force production. Posture is a static indicator of mobility and dynamic movement often exposes compensations in movement patterns and is an indicator of compromised mobility and joint action.

Flexibility

Muscle flexibility is the ability of soft tissues such as muscles, and connective tissues such as tendons and ligaments to lengthen and shorten with higher efficacy, which allows a joint to move through an optimal range of motion because the acting muscle groups have healthy length and tension relationships. In this model, the difference between mobility and flexibility is the value of flexibility may be relative to the application of force and is focused on the muscle, not specifically the joint. For example, a male martial artist may require a unique value of muscular flexibility in some planes versus the needs of a female soccer player.

Stability

Structural stability is simply the encapsulation of joints by properly conditioned stabilization and synergistic muscle groups with higher balance potential, along with a proprioceptive or neuromuscular response. The combination of mobility, flexibility, and stability reduces the risk of injury and improves force production.

Strength

Strength is a word used to define the ability to produce force. More specifically, strength is the ability of a muscle group to generate force at a specified or unchanging velocity. Muscle size is highly correlated to strength, however, other factors such as limb length, and muscle length also determine one's strength.

The word strong is often used to generally describe ones physical ability to lift or move heavy things and this broad definition is fairly accurate. It is important to build a sound base of strength before beginning to train for power.

Power

When we move a given weight over a measured distance and time, we produce power. Power is commonly thought of as explosiveness, and the ability to sprint, jump, and change direction. While great athleticism may be an outcome of power training, power can be realized at slower speeds.

The definition of power is defined as the weight lifted multiplied by the vertical distance traveled, divided by the time to complete the repetition. Using this equation, a person lifting a heavy mass at a slow rate will produce the same amount of power as another person lifting a much lighter mass at a much higher rate. Thus, power in program design is seen in both described methods and it is important to utilize each in program design.

Skill

Skill encompasses the qualities of discipline, motivation, care, and comprehension. The outcome of these characteristics may appear to the eye as coordination, however, do not be fooled, that isn't the only outcome of skill.

Skill is attention to detail repeated consistently and frequently to create the desired adaptation, it is the "it" of fitness training and the X factor that will make or break an exercise. An exerciser becomes highly skilled in an exercise when they can execute the required movements flawlessly with very little mental focus or effort while physical exertion remains high.

This is predominantly seen in advanced weightlifters, athletes, and other performance-based endeavors related to human movement and neuromuscular facilitation.

Acute Variables Basics

Acute variables are simply the design of a program, including load, sets, repetitions, and contraction tempo. For simplicity, I have omitted several acute variables, including training intensity, training volume, rest interval, exercise selection, exercise order, training duration, and training frequency.

To even determine how much to lift and how to lift it, one must first have an accurate picture of their condition level. Because we are very sedentary in the United States, many people have developed compensations in movement patterns and may have altered musculature balance and joint function.

These human movement imbalances result from excessive sitting, hunching, and lack of activity, or even injuries and should be addressed with corrective exercise. Because weight training involves muscle contraction with resistance along the tissue and joint, we are already at great risk of injury when we possess an imbalance.

Lifting too heavy or with the incorrect set of acute variables is likely to place excessive force against the joint and connective tissue such as tendons, ligaments, and fascia. Weight training should be a progressive activity where one takes the time to build strength in joint stabilizer muscles before attempting major prime mover work.

As a basic rule, we should follow the 6 Levels of Fitness Hierarchy when developing a workout program. Here is a considerably basic and common approach for applying acute variables through each phase, according to the National Academy of Sports Medicine:

Weight (load + Intensity)
•Stabilization & Muscle Endurance: 50% – 70% of One Rep Max
•Hypertrophy: 75% – 85% of One Rep Max
•Maximal Strength: 85% – 100% of One Rep Max

Sets (Total Volume of Movement)
•Stabilization & Muscle Endurance: 1 – 3 Sets
•Hypertrophy: 3 – 5 Sets
•Maximal Strength: 4 – 6 Sets

Repetitions: (Time Under Tension)
•Stabilization & Muscle Endurance: 12 – 20 Reps
•Hypertrophy: 6 – 12 Reps
•Maximal Strength: 1 – 5 Reps

Tempo: (Time Under Tension + Maximal Motor Unit Recruitment)

NOTE: In my experience, writing tempo for clients can be extremely confusing on their end so I have found starting with tempo in the first contraction makes more sense. In some applications, the eccentric tempo is displayed first, and this is simply hard to understand for most people who are not personal trainers.

For example, I write a bicep curl with the concentric action to the isometric top end and finally the eccentric back to the isometric start. However, on a squat, the first action is eccentric, but I still write that tempo first as it is the first muscle action.

• Stabilization & Muscle Endurance: 2-3/1-2/3-4
(2-3 second concentric lift, 1-2 second isometric hold, 3-4 second eccentric return)
• Hypertrophy: 2/0/2-3
(2-second concentric lift, 0-second isometric hold, 2-3 second eccentric return)
• Maximal Strength: Explosive concentric and controlled return.

Posture & Form: It's Not How Much, It's How You Lift

Posture is also critical to ensure muscle groups and joints are at their optimal positions to move weight safely and effectively. Posture is the gateway to improving the nervous system and muscle communication and greatly reducing the chances of injury.

Proper posture is fundamental to static (standing or sitting) or dynamic movements (active or athletic) to maintain skeletal alignment, reduce abnormal wearing of joint surfaces, decrease tendon and ligament stress, prevent excessive muscle fatigue, and reduce injuries related to improper movement.

Many postural imbalances become even more pronounced during a dynamic movement and that's exactly when you want to be stable and in proper "form" or posture. This is especially true in a load-bearing activity such as weight training or a deceleration maneuver in a sport.

The best way to think of proper posture in weight training is to avoid any activity which causes you to swing your body to move the weight, arching or rounding your back, lifting your shoulders, jutting your head forward, or locking your knees. This is a sign that the weight is just too heavy, and you cannot safely move it without compensation or the assistance of momentum.

Recovery Basics: Active and Passive Recovery Is Key

Any time we place stress or train any underdeveloped muscle, the result is typically soreness that develops over the next six to twelve hours. Many people new to weight training think soreness is something to fear or a setback in their program. This is true if recovery is not considered in the acute variables of the program design.

On the other hand, muscle soreness is not always an indicator of progress or success in your lifts. As muscles adapt, their soreness quotient diminishes. Tenderness is a natural product of intense resistance or activation of skeletal muscle but must be monitored.

In general, soreness may be more prevalent in a deconditioned person or someone who has intensified their routine, it is a temporary result of weight training and not to be feared. Weight training participants should understand the difference between Delayed Onset Muscle Soreness (DOMS) and overtraining, so check with a fitness professional whenever possible.

Allow the affected tissue time to recover and for the body to mend the muscular tears before working on that muscle group again. This can be done through Passive Recovery by limiting that muscle group's activation over approximately two or three days. Active Recovery is when muscles are stimulated through light stretching, foam rolling, or mild resistance for a period depending on the acute variables of the program.

Recovery must be aligned with your training goal, adequate sleep, and proper nutrition. Recovery time for stabilization exercise is far shorter than the recovery of larger muscle groups and sleep is where most of the full recovery takes place. But of course, nutrition is the bedrock of the whole program. Weight training requires the proper ratio of carbohydrates, proteins, fats, and water to be truly effective, so be sure you have food intake dialed in.

Common Exercise Terms and Modality Basics

I think it's important to tie in some fundamental education about workout types and terms by describing some of the more popular approaches and concepts. The type of workout you choose is greatly dependent on your current condition and goals. Here are the basics of common approaches and fitness terms in alphabetical order:

Active Recovery

Recovery is just as critical as the workouts themselves. Exercise is stress that breaks down muscle through resistance and this needs time to repair. It is the recovery process that finalizes the effort of exercise and improves strength, endurance, and composition.

Active recovery is the method of applying light tension to the muscles in static and dynamic stretching and even self-myofascial release. This facilitates circulation and can speed up recovery and reduce the feelings of soreness.

Aerobic Exercise = With Oxygen

During aerobic exercise, your body utilizes oxygen for energy which is ideal for extended periods of activity. Aerobic modalities include running, walking, cycling rowing, and so forth.

Anaerobic Exercise = Without Oxygen

Anaerobic exercise is any exercise that breaks down glucose in the body without using oxygen. Typically, anaerobic exercises are short and intense. Anaerobic modalities include strength training, HIIT, Tabata, Circuits, sprints, and so forth.

AMRAP = As Many Reps as Possible

AMRAP stands for "As Many Reps as Possible," or conversely, "As Many Rounds as Possible." Either way, you are performing as many reps of a single exercise as you can in a pre-determined period, or as many rounds of several exercises as you can in a pre-determined time.

It is critical to note, that this style of training does not advocate for sloppy form just to get in more work. Never sacrifice the proper form of biomechanical exercise for load or reps. Nothing will derail your progress like an injury.

Circuit Training

Not to be confused with HIIT, Circuit Training is typically done in a systematic selection of weight-based exercises performed in a sequence without rest or at least, truly little. It is usually the combination of at least six or more movements with a set number of rounds and repetition goals. Circuit Training has been shown to improve neuromuscular communication, stability, strength endurance, elevated heart rate, and body composition improvement. Circuits can be broken into hemispherical work such as upper and lower or reciprocal groups of large and smaller support muscles.

Circuit training is a popular approach because it is highly efficient and delivers reasonably predictable results for most practitioners. Those new to weight training or just getting back into workouts may see a favorable return provided the workouts are well constructed and take your current condition into account.

Circuits require careful form and deliberate movements to reduce the risk of injury so be sure you choose a plan that fits your situation or, hire a professional to build a custom plan for you. For the intermediate exerciser, circuits are a fantastic way to change up workouts and move past any plateaus from traditional workout structures.

Circuit Training with Reciprocal Groupings and 3 set Example:

Note: these are two separate workouts that will clock in at about 30-minutes each. You may group them for a total body circuit if you want to increase the time and intensity.

CIRCUIT - CHEST, TRICEPS, SHOULDERS	REPS	TEMPO
Triceps - Dumbbell Overhead Extension	12x	2-1-2
Chest - Dumbbell Press	12x	2-1-2
Shoulder - Dumbbell Lateral Raise	12x	2-1-2
Chest - Dumbbell Fly	12x	2-1-2
Shoulder - Dumbbell Overhead Press	12x	2-1-2
Dumbbell Rear Deltoid Fly	12x	2-1-2
CIRCUIT - BACK, BICEPS, LEGS	REPS	TEMPO
Dumbbell Side Lunge (Left and Right)	12x	2-1-2
Biceps - Dumbbell Curl	12x	2-1-2
Dumbbell Lunge Overhead Press	12x	2-1-2
Dumbbell Standing Row	12x	2-1-2
Goblet Squat	12x	2-1-2
Dumbbell Walking Lunges (Left and Right)	12x	2-1-2

Compound Exercises

Compound exercises activate multiple muscle groups simultaneously. For example, a squat is a compound exercise that works the quadriceps, glutes, and calves and intrinsically activates the core stabilizers. Compound exercises elevate stress and incorporate multiple muscles in a movement for higher levels of efficacy.

Contraction Tempo

The speed at which weight is moved is a major acute variable and fundamental to muscular stress, motor unit recruitment, and adaptation signals. In a professionally constructed workout program, the tempo is indicated by a sequence of 3 numbers. Such as 2-0-2. This is 2 seconds for the contraction or lift, 0 seconds in the middle of the lift, and then 3 seconds to return the weight to the starting position.

The three phases of contraction start with a concentric action followed by isometric contractions and finally eccentric contractions or negatives. Tempo will change based on the intention of the program and should be included in all your workouts. For example, to illicit a power adaptation, your contraction tempo would look like 1-1-1 as you are looking to produce as much force as quickly as possible.

However, a muscle-building or hypertrophy tempo would emphasize more control in the contraction such as 2-0-3/4. You will notice the eccentric action is slow and this is to increase the time the muscle is under tension.

Cool-Down

Incorporating a cool-down in your workout program is critical for optimal recovery and circulatory health. A proper cool-down helps reduce the effect of blood pooling which is a byproduct of elevated heart rate and blood oxygen distribution. If exercise is stopped abruptly, blood can pool in the lower extremities which can make you feel lightheaded or even faint.

It's worth it to take time to allow your circulatory system to stabilize. A cool-down also helps relieve soreness, reduces the risk of injury, and facilitates recovery.

Cross-Training

Cross-training is defined as an exercise program that utilizes several training modalities to develop capacity in several forms of fitness. The typical cross-training program includes resistance training and some form of higher-level aerobic training as well. For example, a marathon runner spends a good deal of their training time running but they often cross-train with resistance to improve overall performance. Cross-training is also ideal for fat loss, muscle retention, and improving overall endurance.

DOMS

Delayed Onset Muscle Soreness can be caused by various types of high-intensity exercise and activities, particularly resistance training. DOMS tends to appear a day or so after a particularly intense or new workout and can last for several days.

When your muscles are exposed to new exercises, higher volume, or weight, they are signaled to work harder than their homeostatic state. This is an increase in stress so you are working past your normal level, and this can cause minor muscle trauma. This is where active recovery is key.

Dynamic Warm-Up

A warm-up prepares you for a workout by increasing blood flow to muscles, raising body temperature, activating metabolic reactions, and improving joint range of motion which reduces the risk of injury.

High-Intensity Interval Training (HIIT).

HIIT is a form of short, intense, and unsustainable surges of activity with strategic rest periods to maximize intensity and recovery. With HIIT, we signal our bodies with metabolic disruption and increase our energy or calorie output in short periods.

Well-constructed HIIT workouts have been shown to improve cardio and pulmonary function, stabilization and balance, muscle endurance, and recruitment plus reduced insulin resistance. HIIT also likely provides additional expenditure of energy because of a phenomenon called Excess-Post Exercise Oxygen Consumption (EPOC), which for the sake of brevity we will not detail in this book.

This modality is also popular because it does not require any special equipment, takes less time to complete, and delivers results for most practitioners. HIIT is an approach that is ideal to supplement strength training and can be done one to four times each week for generally healthy individuals.

High-Intensity Interval Training Example:

EXERCISE ORDER – PERFORM 3 ROUNDS	DURATION	REST
Burpee	45 Seconds	15 Seconds
Squat Jump	45 Seconds	15 Seconds
Sumo squat pulse	45 Seconds	15 Seconds
Hollow Body Hold	45 Seconds	15 Seconds
Sit Up	45 Seconds	15 Seconds
Bicycle Crunch	45 Seconds	15 Seconds
Plank to Push Up	45 Seconds	15 Seconds
Cross Body Mountain Climber	45 Seconds	15 Seconds
Glute Bridge	45 Seconds	15 Seconds
Body Weight Alternating Jump Lunge	45 Seconds	15 Seconds
Jumping Jack	45 Seconds	15 Seconds
Running in Place	45 Seconds	15 Seconds
Push-Up	45 Seconds	15 Seconds
Burpee Squat Thrust	45 Seconds	15 Seconds
Wall Sit	45 Seconds	15 Seconds

Isometric Training

Isometric exercises are isolated exercises where you contract a muscle or muscle group and hold it in a fixed position for the duration of the exercise. An example would be a plank, hollow body hold, or low squat hold.

Loading Horizontal and Vertical

Loading is simply the value of the weight used in each exercise. Horizontal loading is considered the classic approach. In this load structure, you complete the first set of an exercise and then rest before you execute the next set of the same exercise. You can have as many sets as needed for your particular goal, but rest and repetitions should be considered to ensure your adaption outcome is what you are intending.

On the other hand, vertical loading is like a circuit. Essentially, you execute one movement and move on to the next exercise with minimal or no rest. Once you get to the end of your outlined exercises, you start back at the top with the first exercise. Vertical loading can be anywhere between one to four sets and is generally done by moving from lowers to uppers or vice versa within the set.

Plyometric Training

Plyometric training is a form of intense movements that involve explosive contraction and eccentrically focused deceleration. Ideal for athletes or those looking to improve their multi-planar functionality, plyometrics improves speed, power, and force production.

Reps or Repetitions

Reps are the number of times you complete a single exercise before resting in a set. Rep ranges differ based on your desired outcome so be sure your rep range is aligned with your goal.

Rate of Perceived Exertion

The RPE is used by trainers to determine the estimated rate of exertion. You can use this basic scale to determine the approximate intensity of an exercise. While the Borg Scale is the clinical approach, most people find it confusing so simply rate your work on a scale of one through ten. One of course is super easy and ten being extremely hard.

Sets

A set is the number of cycles you complete in a workout. Each set is comprised of reps. Your set and rep range should be set based on your adaptation goal and adjusted frequently to avoid plateaus in your progress.

Set Variation – Straight Sets

This is the most common method for designing a resistance training program set system. Straight sets are performed using the same number of repetitions, weight, tempo, and rest within the set group.

Set Variation – Drop Sets

This set approach is a unique way to increase muscle fatigue and improve composition but is not commonly used in performance training. A drop set is where you start your first set and push the load to form failure within a certain rep range. Then, without rest, you reduce the weight and execute the next set again to form failure.

Set Variation – Compound Sets

This set structure is nearly identical to the superset system but lacks variety. This is because compound sets specifically mean working the same muscles with two different exercises in one set.

Set Variation – Pyramid Sets

This set structure is based on the approach of gradually increasing the intensity of your lifts by adding to the load each set but reducing the repetitions in the next set.

Steady-State Cardio

Steady-state cardio is simply any continuous cardio workout, steady effort, as opposed to an interval cardio workout where you vary your energy output. While steady state has its place in endurance training, it is not considered optimal for fat loss compared to other modalities such as intervals.

Supersets

Super setting means pairing two or more exercises and executing them back-to-back without rest. Supersets are efficient means of exercising because you can save time by working on two different muscle groups together, so you eliminate rest between the superset exercise and get more time under tension.

With a traditional superset, one muscle group is recovering while the other is still working. However, you can superset with opposing muscles, synergistic muscles, closed-chain movements, open-chain movements, and various load patterns such as drop sets or vertical loads.

Supersets can increase the activation of multiple muscle groups, streamline workouts, reduce the time of exercise, and increase heart rate. Be sure your contraction tempo is set per your intended outcome.

Superset Training Example:
Note: This is a total body basic superset that clocks in at about 45-55 minutes. Unlike a circuit, you complete all three sets of the two exercises before moving on to the next group of movements. The rest is only after both exercises are complete within that set.

EXERCISE ORDER – PERFORM 3 SETS	REPS	TEMPO
Biceps - Dumbbell Curl	12	2-0-2
Back - Dumbbell Standing Row	12	2-0-2
REST 45-60 Seconds		
Legs - Dumbbell Straight Leg Deadlift	12	2-0-2
Legs - Kettlebell Goblet Squat	12	2-0-2
REST 45-60 Seconds		
Bicep - Dumbbell Hammer Curl	12	2-0-2
Shoulder - Dumbbell Rear Deltoid Fly	12	2-0-2
REST 45-60 Seconds		
Legs - Sumo Squat Pulse	12	2-0-2
Legs - Sumo Glute Bridge	12	2-0-2
REST 45-60 Seconds		
Chest – Dumbbell Press	12	2-0-2
Triceps – Overhead Extension	12	2-0-2
REST 45-60 Seconds		
Shoulder – Dumbbell Overhead Press	12	2-0-2
Shoulder – Dumbbell Lateral Raise	12	2-0-2

Traditional Strength Training

Strength training includes forms of resistance to stress your muscle and may include dumbbells, kettlebells, barbells, or cables.

Traditional Hypertrophy Training Example:

Note: This is a split system where the muscles are broken down into a synergistic grouping of three muscles. These kinds of workouts used here as an example should not be done together but done 2-3 times each week to introduce adequate stress and recovery for muscular development. It is also recommended that you lift at least 70% of your max in the beginning and then increase weight over time as you adapt. You may also need to organize the order of exercises based on your biofeedback. Some people prefer to do the big lifts first such as the deadlift and back squat so they can lift heavier on those movements. Finally, this is not a circuit, and all sets of an exercise should be performed before you move on to the next one.

BACK, BICEPS & LEGS – PERFORM 3 SETS	REPS	TEMPO
Back - Cable Seated Close Grip Row	6-8	2-0-3
REST 60-90 Seconds		
Biceps - Dumbbell Bicep Curl	6-8	2-0-3
REST 60-90 Seconds		
Legs – Barbell Back Squat	6-8	2-0-3
REST 60-90 Seconds		
Back - Lat Machine Wide Grip Pulldown	6-8	2-0-3
REST 60-90 Seconds		
Biceps - Dumbbell Hammer Curl	6-8	2-0-3
REST 60-90 Seconds		
Legs - Barbell Deadlift	6-8	2-0-3
REST 60-90 Seconds		
Back – Reverse Fly	6-8	2-0-3
REST 60-90 Seconds		
Biceps – Close Grip EZ Curl Bar	6-8	2-0-3
REST 60-90 Seconds		

Legs - Machine Leg Press	6-8	2-0-3
CHEST, TRICEPS & SHOULDERS – PERFORM 3 SETS	**REPS**	**TEMPO**
Triceps - Cable Extension	6-8	2-0-3
REST 60-90 Seconds		
Chest - Dumbbell Press	6-8	2-0-3
REST 60-90 Seconds		
Shoulder - Dumbbell Overhead Press	6-8	2-0-3
REST 60-90 Seconds		
Triceps - Cable Reverse Grip Pulldown	6-8	2-0-3
REST 60-90 Seconds		
Chest - Standing Cable Fly	6-8	2-0-3
REST 60-90 Seconds		
Shoulder – Dumbbell Later Raise	6-8	2-0-3
REST 60-90 Seconds		
Triceps – Dumbbell Overhead Extension	6-8	2-0-3
REST 60-90 Seconds		
Chest – Dumbbell Incline with Crush Grip	6-8	2-0-3
REST 60-90 Seconds		
Shoulder – Alternating Dumbbell Frontal Raise	6-8	2-0-3

5 Reasons Women Should Be Weight Training

All right, this is a subject I am passionate about, and I will be very direct. Somehow, someway, our society has placed women in the cardio section and men in the weight room. I wholeheartedly encourage all women to turn off the treadmill, get down from the stair climber and stop wasting time on the elliptical trainer and add strength training into their programs.

I am not saying cardio is bad or that you should not be doing some form of cardio. It is a critical component to balanced fitness, such as vascular and pulmonary health. Here are five reasons women need to be strength training:

One – Weight training will increase your strength and improve your overall functionality as a mother, spouse, caregiver, athlete, professional or in any other capacity you can apply enhanced strength advantages. Strength transcends just muscle action or power.

We have ligaments, tendons, fascia, stabilizing, and synergistic muscle groups that all benefit from proper strength training. This means the very fabric of your body gets stronger, more durable, and resistant to injury.

Proper weight training increases positive hormonal response, cellular regeneration, connective tissue health, and your capacity to do work. Essentially, structured strength training upgrades your body and optimizes your functionality.

Two – Resistance training improves heart health and if you did not know, the number one killer of women in the United States is heart disease. We are talking about triglyceride management, cholesterol, blood pressure, resting heart rate, heart rate recovery, not to mention arterial, vinous, and capillary efficiency, and health.

Cardio also helps in this regard, but most ladies are stuck in steady-state cardio sessions, and instead of increasing intensity to get out of a plateau, most women just increase duration. This is a common and serious mistake.

You need to change your intensity levels, not necessarily duration unless you are an endurance athlete with a properly constructed training schedule. Why would you add time to workouts and not focus on the best activities for return on that investment and improve your heart health?

Three - Bone density is a major problem for many countries where starvation is a factor in the formative years, such as puberty. Yet Americans always find a way to have everything and nothing. We are so overfed and have access to all sorts of fancy medical gimmicks and procedures but can't even keep proper bone health because of poor nutritional choices, not starvation, and because we are outrageously sedentary.

Ladies of all ages, you do not need to suffer from excessive bone loss as you age, even after menopause. It is usually a self-imposed condition and strength training will improve your bone density and health. Now I get it, everyone jumps to age, genetics, or family history instantly, especially if the solution requires effort.

But we are talking about a small percentage of women that are predisposed to chronic bone wasting. Even light resistance training three to four times each week can dramatically improve bone health. Strength training also improves coordination and neuromuscular efficiency, so you are less likely to fall, to begin with.

Four – Lean muscle helps reduce body fat and fat accumulation. Now, I am speaking in terms of good health and not aesthetics, I will get to that in point five. Lean muscle elevates your metabolism, especially when in a constant or structured state of contraction because it requires energy.

Our bodies get energy from calories, and if you have a strong, balanced, and measured nutritional lifestyle and are active, your body does not need excess fat. Lean muscle and appropriate levels of caloric intake nearly always provide a positive metabolic response.

Five – Muscle makes women look amazing. Strong is beautiful and historically, women have been physically strong until we got soft with our cushy modern conveniences. I will say it plain, ladies, you have been lied to. Muscle is not masculine, it is human. You can't get "bulky" with well-structured light or moderate weightlifting, heck most guys can't even gain muscle easily!

You do not have the hormonal or biological makeup to be overly muscular. I concede a potential genetic factor can cause some women to be larger in some body parts than others or have a heavier frame, but this should be celebrated, not feared.

Women are supposed to have curves and some muscle definition as indicated by their very own physiology. Ladies, you look amazing with muscle. Yes, by density compared to fat, muscle takes up less space than the equivalent weight of fat, so ignore the scale. Throw it away and focus on your lean muscle volume and lower your total percentage of body fat.

Remember, strength training holds you together, improves cardiac function, boosts metabolism and hormonal health, increases bone density, and makes you look fantastic. Work from the inside out and that is where you find fitness joy.

3 Reasons to Stop Weighing Yourself Frequently

Weighing yourself every day or a few times each week is counterproductive and not, by any means, an effective or objective system for validating fat loss. There are several factors here and I will start with my favorite soapbox: the media, fitness industry, unscrupulous trainers, and fitness product manufacturers have altered reasonable expectations for results as it relates to the timeframe and effort required.

In addition, our parents and grandparents have done one hell of a job emotionally tying our self-image and, ultimately, self-worth to the meaningless number on a scale. Even my beloved late grandmother was a body weight tyrant to me, my siblings, and my mom. This is how she was raised, and it transferred.

We have created this fake set of "acceptable" weights based on arbitrary numbers and without taking any other external conditions into account. While your body weight is a factor, it is not the defining factor nor the ultimate objective system for measuring your physique or even fitness level. Here are three reasons the scale is not helping you.

One - Muscle, by volume, is approximately five times denser than fat. This means that when you take five pounds of fat, it is around the size of a football where five pounds of muscle is around the size of a softball. That is a huge difference when considered from an anatomical distribution standpoint.

Muscle is lean, looks great, and has outstanding health benefits. On the other hand, fat is flabby, unsightly, and has negative health consequences. As I pointed out in the last section, one of the greatest fitness injustices historically has been the notion women should not lift weights. Women are so emotionally bonded to a scale, for no practical reason at all, and this must end.

Yes, some men are emotionally bound to the scale, but it seems less dramatic. Women need strength training just as much and if not more than men as they age. Adding muscle will likely increase your total weight, but you will be strong, lithe, fit, aesthetically pleasing, and boost your metabolism.

Who cares how much you weigh? The scale will lie to you about your composition. Build muscle, burn fat, ditch the scale, and measure the total percentage of body fat and worry less about your weight.

Two – As far as objective assessment of your results and physique are concerned, body circumference measurements are superior. The scale only tells one side of the story yet measuring the girth of key body parts such as the neck, shoulders, arms, chest, waist, hips, and thigh gives you a much better and useful picture as it relates to your composition. If you have a good starting measurement, then you can always compare over time and see your results in vivid contrast.

Conversely, if you are not seeing the results you expect, you know that you need to rapidly adjust your nutrition or workout program. Measurements validate your efforts and provide a highly personalized reference point that is exclusive to you. I recommend taking body circumference measurements over scales any day.

If you want to learn how to take these measurements, just go to the Forge YouTube channel. I have a video there that gives you a detailed step-by-step on how to take them.

Three – The scale does not show you how much better you are feeling or how your clothes are getting loose. The scale does not show you lower LDL cholesterol, triglycerides, or blood glucose. The scale will not show you energy, endurance, or positive hormonal response to proper nutrition and elevated activity levels. The scale will not give you compliments, like a friend or family member who could see the subtle changes you are blind to.

In summary, the scale is more damaging than constructive. It only gives you a narrow view and partial representation of your progress and the downside is significantly more than the upside. I encourage all my clients, and now the readers of this book, to be objective about your fitness and progress.

Use a measurement system like circumference or total body fat percentage compared to lean mass instead of total body weight. It gives you a clear picture and gets you out of the programmed negativity relate to the scale.

Top 5 Mistakes People Make at The Gym

In this segment, I would like to reiterate my deep empathy for those struggling to make fitness a part of their lives. I understand how hard it can be to overcome the fear of gyms, the perception of judgment, or the feeling of not knowing what you are doing. However, there are some common holes that so many people fall into, and I intend to expose the challenges and offer solutions.

I am not outlining the Top 5 Mistakes People Make at The Gym to be antagonistic. But my goodness people, some of the things I see are silly and quite easily avoided with some common sense. I find it fascinating when people are surprised after they miss half their workouts each week for a month and get upset because they did not see results. Then some show up to the gym, but they are not doing the work.

Workouts are ended early, the weight lifted is too light or they simply sit on a bike barely pedaling while reading a gossip magazine. But what if you are focused and hitting each workout as hard as you are able and still, no results? It happens and when it does, go back to the planning phase and evaluate your program. Are the sets, reps, tempo, rest intervals, weight, frequency, volume, modality, and duration appropriate for your goal?

Mistake One: Expecting Instant Results

Expecting instant results is the number one mistake because it sets the stage for all the other mistakes we make regarding fitness and nutrition. This ties back into the "Duration Lie" I exposed in the first chapter.

Where is my soapbox? Ah, here it is: There are two problems here. First, in our culture of instant gratification, people are less inclined to put forth the effort. We are often lazy, deconditioned, and have an endless stream of excuses for our state of body and mind. Plus, we expect an instant return on most everything. Consider how quickly we can even get information. No more library because we can quickly retrieve info from a website or search engine. We are trained to want it now.

Second, the media has done a remarkable job creating false hope, producing gimmicks, and generating fads designed to sell you crappy products that promise to deliver on our hyper-focus for instant gratification. Even unethical Doctors and unprofessional Personal Trainers use words like" magic," "miracle" or "fountain of youth" to sell products. We see infomercials and testimonials from people that claim they easily lost 30 pounds in 30 days simply by taking the latest miracle pill.

Or they claim your dreams come true if you eat a highly specialized diet that, of course, requires you to buy some kind of "magic" shake, coffee, oil, butter, lotion, vibrating pad, sweat wrap, or other such nonsense. Then some go all-in with the super extreme way and remove parts of your digestive system with banding, bypasses, and other cosmetically focused augmentation to avoid the tedious and seemingly unreasonable approach of proper nutrition and physical activity.

How insane is that? We would prefer to remove body parts rather than stop eating poor-quality food and taking a walk each day. Here is the truth, none of the things I just mentioned have made a dent in our declining health as a nation. They do not work. They are not sustainable and do not address the root cause. The only way to safely and effectively improve your fitness is to change your habits, eat properly, exercise and repeat.

Women, you should only be losing 1 or 1.5 pounds per week when working towards fat loss. Men, you might be able to lose 2 pounds each week safely. It is so easy to eat 3,500 calories in a day, but to burn it off can take a week. Now I know some people can lose more than others and some are even successful at sustaining it, but that is the exception, not the rule. Just because someone won the lottery, does not mean you will win it next by buying one ticket. It's a fallacy and we must examine our expectations and adjust to reality.

Let's take a step back from the chaos of marketing and the propaganda that fuels these unrealistic expectations for how long it will take to meet your fitness desires. Each of us must take personal responsibility and acknowledge that fitness and food management are everyday occurrences.

We must take responsibility for our health and that of our children, considering 35% of adults and nearly 20% of children are morbidly obese in our country. That is not including those that are "overfat" which is 7 out of 10 Americans. Once you get your expectations aligned, then you can set up your program for success.

Mistake Two: Failing to Plan, Schedule, and Track workouts.

If we want to nitpick, then we could even say there are three mistakes here, but to keep this simple, we combine them because they are all related to the initial program design. I have always been surprised by how a vast majority of new exercisers or novice gym-goers ignore the critical concept of developing a simple and realistic plan that is scheduled and tracked. The saying goes: "if you fail to plan, you plan to fail."

I also get disappointed when people claim they don't know what to do or where to start. And it is not completely their fault. I understand this because the amount of fitness opinion, content, and media is overwhelming. The fitness industry and media have sensationalized fitness to the point people become confused or fear they will choose the wrong path, thus wasting time and even money.

This is also true for diets. I say to you, the first thing is to clear the clutter and focus on the very basics. First, create a simple total body resistance and cardio plan based on your current condition while keeping your goal in mind. Second, create a balanced and nutritionally dense meal plan by reigning in calories and omitting processed foods and poor sources that accommodate the needs of your activity level and goal.

Let's break fitness into planning, scheduling, and tracking. When you write your plan, look at it objectively and see if you address some important aspects such as injury, mobility issues, and what equipment you have available. For optimum health, you must engage in intensity-appropriate resistance and cardio training several times each week.

If you are not comfortable with strength training or have never lifted weights, then I recommend you hire a professional trainer to show you, and don't be cheap. If it matters to you, then invest in yourself. Consider your gym peak times and class schedules if you would like to avoid the rush and maximize your workouts or reduce the intimidation factor.

Once you design a plan that looks good, it's time to execute it. The best way to start this is to schedule your workouts for each day and walk through the gym door with a specific and measurable plan. You can schedule on a mobile device and set alarms or go to traditional paper. Also, plan the schedule to accommodate commute traffic, work projects, and family obligations.

If you do not make time for and schedule your workouts, you will likely slip back into an old habitual schedule or ignore the intention of your plan. A scheduled workout is simply a documented promise to yourself. And finally, track your workouts diligently. This not only helps focus in the gym and engage with your process, but it also will help identify what is or is not working in your plan.

All workout plans should be written for approximately four to six weeks to illicit the General Adaptation Syndrome, which is the point at which you reach a plateau. At that point, you must modify your plan to move past that point and inspire the body to further adapt. When I say adapt or adaptation, I mean results. Plateaus are good, but only if you know how to get past and into the next adaptation phase.

Again, this is where hiring a professional makes a huge difference. I believe everyone must take personal responsibility and learn more about their body and the science of exercise and nutrition. Our world has changed with the rapid introduction of technological conveniences, and we are so sedentary, keeping a lean frame and getting in enough activity requires a whole new lifestyle. Yes, it's complex, yet everyone needs to know the basics in our modern world of sitting and fast food.

Mistake Three: Getting Stuck in a Plateau.

This may be new information for many people, but a dirty word in fitness is "routine." If you have ever maintained a fitness program for any reasonable period, you have experienced a plateau. Most people see a weight loss or strength plateau as a negative, yet it is quite the opposite and a sign your body has adapted to the "stress" of your exercise program. This means that what you were doing worked and your body made specific adaptations to the demand of your workouts.

This is where we see measurable results. Yet many people become frustrated and do not know how to get the body to respond to further illicit results or what fitness professionals call "adaptations" let's briefly dive into the science so you will have a better understanding of what your body is going through physiologically and be better equipped to get past this temporary phase of a plateau. I will keep this simple and abridged.

We already touched on the General Adaptation Syndrome in earlier chapters. It is the predictable way the body restores itself to balance, or homeostasis, in response to stress. While there are applications of the adaptation syndrome beyond fitness, I am going to only focus on the three stages as they relate to how we get into and then break plateaus.

The first phase of this adaptation process is "The Alarm Stage" and is the initial response when stress is first recognized by the body. The autonomic nervous system activates the sympathetic response, or the fight or flight effect, which is a hormonal response rooted in survival. We have all experienced that adrenaline rush when someone jumps out and scares us. Our bodies immediately release hormones, including cortisol, adrenaline, and noradrenaline. Adrenaline immediately raises the blood pressure and heart rate, so we can react. When the stress is removed, the body returns to normal. In exercise, it is the physiological stress of resistance and elevated activity outside of our homeostasis that causes the alarm.

Next is the "Resistance Stage" or in a more direct description, the adaptation phase. In this stage, the body adjusts its structures or enzyme levels to grant protection against stress, specifically exercise. The type of training you are performing determines the type of adaptation. This is the reason for the "specificity" of the adaptive response in your training and why "Acute Variables" such as set, reps, tempo, rest, load, and frequency are so important to have nailed down. One way to avoid frustration over the lack of results is to train for your goal. For example, in a strength training session, you signal a specific output and cellular response in tissues involved in producing strength. The stimulation of these cells during a strength training session will dictate the type of structural changes during recovery to make the cell stronger for the next training session. Activation of the immune system strengthens the defense capacity of the body and stimulates the repair process by dismantling and rebuilding damaged cells.

Now here is where it gets tricky because too much "stress" and you go into the "Exhaustion Phase," but if you do not have enough stress or intensity in your workouts, then you will likely not optimally provoke your body into the desired adaptation. Essentially, you need to have the right acute variables around your program to get the return on your investment of time and energy. But applying too much stress may cause you to enter the exhaustion phase and you may feel fatigued and irritable. The body runs out of reserve energy and stress affects your mental, physical, and emotional stability.

When excessive long-term stress persists, as in the case of overtraining, you will stop seeing results and will need to take forced recovery. The purpose of training is to cause the body to adapt to specific stressors and produce "results" such as mobility, stability, strength, power, and neuromuscular skill. Training should strengthen physiological systems, activate the correct energy systems, and repair damaged cells.

Train based on your current level of condition and goal and always incorporate the recovery time as a part of your program. Train at the right intensity and ensure you get adequate rest and recovery. Not too much rest or you can de-train or go backward and conversely, too much intensity and you go into the exhaustion phase.

Mistake Four: Using Weight Loss as A Primary Goal.

It may sound counterintuitive, but let's be realistic about this and objectively consider the following. If your body composition, or weight, was that important, then you would never let yourself become overweight, to begin with. We have proven repeatedly that our appearance is typically not enough to inspire fitness, food management, or a focused behavior improvement for the long term.

It's not like we woke up one morning, looked in the mirror, and said, "Wow! Where did these 50 pounds come from?" We see the weight accumulating but for some reason or another, we do little or nothing until it reaches a tipping point. In general, people who use weight or aesthetics as a primary motivator typically are in the gain-lose-gain-lose-gain cycle. It's time to break that cycle. But why does this trend of an overweight population persist?

It is because the consequences of poor lifestyle choices and excessive weight gain are delayed and gradual. For example, we all know smoking cigarettes is detrimental to health. Yet millions of people still smoke. My question is, what if smoking one cigarette immediately gave you lung cancer? Who would smoke? Aside from the awful reality of addiction, smokers smoke because of instant gratification and delayed consequences. Plain and simple.

Food addiction is similar because you get a dopamine release, and there are no instant consequences, at least in our minds. However, the consequences are profoundly cumulative and like all drugs, breaking the addiction is hard.

To break the cycle of food abuse and workout neglect, you must reform your habits and think long-term. What kind of goals or motivators are realistic? First, you must make the conscious, honest, and committed decision to change. Let's talk about 5 quick goal examples that hold more power than your body image:

Set goals intended to optimize your health and quality of life

This means you must delay instant gratification and think about the long term. How do you want to function at 65, 75, 85, or even 100 years of age? In your mind, what will the end of your life look like? Will you be bedridden with diabetes, heart disease, or other debilitating illnesses brought around by your decisions years ago? Or will you be spry, strong, and active?

Set goals based on a physical activity

This includes activities such as an epic hike, snow sports, water sports, mud runs, cycling, 5k events, or even a marathon or triathlon. When you incorporate these kinds of activities into your life, you are creating a "lifestyle," and your food and fitness follow.

Set goals external to your person

If you have family or children, set an example of personal responsibility or health, and ensure the quality of time spent with them. Don't be the overweight parent or any parent, for that matter, that has overweight kids because you trained them to follow your poor choices and transferred your sedentary life and food addiction. Make the health of your family a goal.

Set goals that improve the way you feel mentally and physically

There are few feelings in the world like having a body and mind that can withstand stress, activity, or even injury. Managing our whole being is attractive in professional and personal arenas. I'm not talking about composition; I'm talking about constitution.

Set goals that inspire others

Get outside of yourself and be a support to your family, career peers, and community. When you humbly live by example, then others aspire to duplicate your success. This doesn't mean you get to brag about your over-the-top fad diet within 37 seconds of meeting someone or explicitly outline the merits of CrossFit. I'm not talking about the fad monsters. I'm talking about a humble example that people see and feel from you, not what you tell them. Set goals that inspire others.

Mistake Five: Comparing Yourself to Others

I have found over the years people are shocked to learn that as a fitness professional, I view this to be an egregious mistake. I will break my reasoning down into 3 primary components.

First, there is nothing wrong with some healthy competition when it comes to relatively even playing fields. For example, when the merit, skill, or discipline where two individuals have the potential to produces equal results, then competition is great. It motivates, creates camaraderie, and boosts personal performance.

For example, if two athletes are competing in a sport, we can assume they have approximately the same skill, training, and opportunity to succeed. While genetic potential is a factor, the field is still relatively even. That is what makes these competitions so exciting to watch. Two prime athletes are battling over milliseconds or inches.

However, the general population is not competing at that level. We are not reaching our genetic potential, nor do we focus nearly exclusively on our workouts or nutrition to optimize performance. We are in different stages of life and the gym floor is not an even field. We have mobility problems, injury, time restraints, family and professional obligations, resources disparity, knowledge, and differing goals.

Comparing oneself to the professional figure competitor in the weight room is a quick way to get frustrated and intimidated to paralysis. They have two or more hours daily to work out and are sponsored or paid to do it. You likely have forty or sixty minutes and other obligations.

Second, something that has disturbed me over the years as it relates to the fitness industry is the before and after picture fallacy. I have a fundamental problem with using other people's before and after photos for sales or motivation. Gyms, trainers, and other fitness or weight loss product manufacturers use pictures of people who may or may not have any relevant comparison to yourself. I feel using these pictures is manipulative and is usually accompanied by ridiculous claims of fantastical results in absurd amounts of time.

They are used to get consumers to believe the product will work for them just like it did for the other "real" people in these before and after photos. Unfortunately, a good portion of these photos are false or not telling the whole story. These photos tie into mistakes one and four, which are expecting instant results and using weight loss or body image as a primary goal or motivation. Mistakes one, four, and five are all related to and reinforced by each other.

Finally, humans come in a large range of height, weight, structures, and conditions. We are not created equal. We have endomorphic, mesomorphic, and ectomorphic body types. We have a genetic predisposition for fat distribution, disease, or other conditions. We have limitations of resources, time and even our personalities can dictate to what degree we aspire in fitness.

Comparing yourself to others is by no means a proactive or positive way to assess your fitness or body composition. This simply means that when you add the sum of your lifestyle, you should be the best you can be, so you feel and even look your best. Focus on yourself and compare to your photo progress. I even encourage all my clients to do this, so we can be objective about ourselves.

If you look at a picture of yourself three months ago and don't like what you see, change it. Make the decision, create a plan and course correct your life. Conversely, if you are happy with a picture of yourself three months ago and want to take it to the next level, then do so. But don't get stuck in the trap of comparing yourself to others. It does not matter. The only thing that matters is you. How do you feel? How do you look? Do you like the course of your life? Are you mastering your habits?

Chapter Fifteen
OVERCOMING FEELINGS OF DEFEAT

I would like to share with you five simple steps to get yourself out of a psychological rut when you are feeling defeated, tired, or simply overwhelmed with life challenges. No doubt this is an issue that we all face, whether it's in fitness, professional career, or personal life. As an example, I will share with you a message from a client because I feel like all of us have been in the situation she describes.

Her message serves as a great example of how many of us often feel. I will share the five steps I sent her in response. She's an amazing woman, so with just this little bit of support, she's been able to keep on the program and enjoy the benefit of several fitness milestone achievements. Here's what she wrote:

"Hey, Michael. I know I've missed my workouts so far this week. With my husband being down with this flu I am pulling double duty at home while still trying to recover myself, and of course, the last two days have been completely overwhelming at work, and I am struggling just to find a few minutes to eat my meals and get my workouts in.

I promise I am trying – tomorrow is a new day, and another shot at getting it right. I had a little breakdown today and had a soda. As I was wondering why the heck I was drinking it, I think I realized that when I get so overwhelmed and stressed, and I feel like I am out of control, ironically I grab something unhealthy because I want to and somehow fulfilling a want for myself seems like some kind of an achievement which gives me a feeling of control.

It's ironic because it's completely the opposite. If I were in control, I would just grab a glass of water since that fits with my goals. It's been a rough couple of days. Any advice for getting back on the horse when you're feeling overwhelmed and a little defeated?"

The feelings she described are common and even I struggle with getting back on my program if I fall off for a couple of days. I also would tell you nine out of ten people have the same issue with food or finding a quick source of fulfillment. One thing I can say with certainty is that I have observed throughout the years working as a fitness professional: Overcoming these feelings does not require a complex neuro-psycho pattern solution.

With modern fitness programming, it comes down to the simplicity of execution and an elevated Wellness Consciousness we covered in part one of this book. The more direct and clearly defined a process is for people with a busy schedule, the easier it is to adopt them into a daily function. I like to avoid over-complicating processes because they become prohibitive. Meaning that people will be less likely to sustain best practices that can improve or enhance their fitness levels if we remove the practical application. Here are super simple steps to walk yourself through when you feel defeated, tired, or tempted. 5 steps to overcoming feelings of defeat:

Stop and Acknowledge

Stop and acknowledge how you are feeling so you can be objective about what's happening in your life and the conditions that may influence your feelings. By pausing for a moment and summing up your situation, you will be mindful and gain a better perspective for decision-making. This is the Power of Conscious Response.

Set Micro Goals

Make a quick and attainable goal for the moment or that same day and then go accomplish it. Something simple like a plank for sixty seconds or ten pushups are good micro-goals because they take less than one minute and the act of doing a quick exercise changes your state.

Plus, you can find sixty seconds somewhere in your schedule to create a small success. It's also important to remember that in fitness, success is cumulative. This means that even what would be defined as a moderate or small success compounds and adds to your collective accomplishment.

Enjoy the Journey

Remind yourself this is a journey and not all paths are smooth and easy-going. It's ok to have bumps along the way because that makes each milestone a super success and gives it meaning. For example, don't focus on the 50, 60, 70, or even 80 lbs you want to shed but focus on the 2, 5, or 8 pounds.

Take it one step at a time, and suddenly, the rough patches of the journey are not so hard because they are what make it worth it in the end. That's why it is such an accomplishment when you get to the top. Remember, mountains are climbed one step at a time.

Recount Your Success

If you know that a workout will be missed and it's unavoidable, be careful not to get frustrated or down on yourself. Instead, resolve to make up that workout when you can. Keep a positive mindset by reminding your psyche of the big picture and reflect on how great you have been doing. Recount how much stronger you are in a plank or how the HIIT is not as challenging because you are getting better.

Control Your Reactions

Remember that one thing you control is how you react to your situation. It is hard and takes practice to master your responses or feelings but project to the next day. In the morning, will you feel better or worse if you make the wrong food choice or decide to skip a workout? For most people, it's not the act of having a soda or skipping workouts that start the cycle of failure. It's the next day when the regret kicks in or they feel like all the previous work was for nothing. Some people even say at this point, it's just too hard to change, so they miserably stay in their comfort zone. But it's a trap, not a comfort zone. So, fight it and get free! Start the next day with even more determination and it will pay off.

Chapter Sixteen
OVERCOMING FITNESS FAILURE

The term "failure" should swiftly be replaced by the word "lesson" when you possess the sense to recognize and alter personal behavior to avoid repeating a mistake in the future. We should only define actions as a true failure when we stop trying to improve. If you do not possess the sense to recognize a reoccurring learning opportunity presented by your unsuccessful actions, that is true failure.

Therefore, when you have a worthy goal, a personal expectation, or a milestone to which you aspire, be resolute and stay the course with determined integrity. Endure the pressure of each challenge and overcome the moments of second-guessing. Never give up. Just today, thousands of Americans are stepping on scales or looking in mirrors wondering what happened. In many cases, people feel worse year-over-year and are in a state of chronic health decline.

These people are experiencing yet another fitness failure and become frustrated, discouraged, and, in some severe cases, depressed. We have so many rational excuses such as family, career, time, or even injuries we can point to, but at the end of it all, we are stuck in the cycle.

Here are 5 specific support-based exercise actions you can take while working on your behavior transformation to make the health and physique composition change you seek attainable and permanent:

Select and Hire a Professional Personal Trainer or Coach.

Without question, the ideal track to sustainable success is investing in a personal trainer. And yes, you can afford it if you truly want to make a permanent lifestyle change. Money is important, but not as critical as your wellness. Not to mention, online personal training or coaching has become a fantastic alternative to live-personal training.

Online options are very affordable by comparison, and there are some excellent advantages to virtual training. In any case, a good personal trainer or coach will design a comprehensive program based on your current condition and goal. They will progressively structure workouts and evaluate progress periodically to measure results. All you must do is show up two or three times each week and execute the workout under their guidance.

You must also perform any other exercise or programs they prescribe to complete on your own. Training in-person with a real professional may cost you between $500 – $1,000 each month and is usually worth it if you find the right trainer. Online options vary and so will the quality of workout programming, communication, and support technology. But not all trainers, virtual or otherwise, are a fit for everyone. Online training can range from $50 – $600 per month depending on the company, trainer, and program.

Join A Small Group Training Program.

Aside from private personal training, working in a group is an excellent way to get involved with a community of others seeking the same change as yourself. This gives you a network of supporters and a strong degree of positive accountability. Plus, small group training can be very affordable and allow you to maximize your budget and time. Remember, small group training should have less than ten participants to be optimal.

Too often, fitness clubs try and cram as many people into a "small" group as possible to drive revenue. I find this unacceptable as a fitness professional and encourage you to seek programs with integrity and solid programming. In a small group setting, a professional trainer can give you a good deal of attention and keep you working safely and effectively. Again, a worthwhile trainer or fitness facility will charge a fair price and you get what you pay for. Don't be cheap with your health and fitness because it just adds to discouragement, poor results, and lost cash. Find a company offering groups of 6-10 that run classes two or three times per week and be prepared to spend between $10- $25 per session.

Get Involved with Group Exercise Classes.

Not to be confused with small group training, a Group Exercise class is a regularly scheduled and pre-formatted fitness class led by an instructor. Classes like these are a great way to get connected to the fitness community, make acquaintances, and enhance your enjoyment of working out. Group classes are a fantastic way to supplement a workout program or personal training session by adding variety and some social components.

Fitness is a journey and having others around you sharing positive energy and enthusiasm goes a long way toward sustainability. Most national brand gyms offer these classes, yet I am inclined to seek smaller or boutique programs as they have a very high level of quality control and instructor oversight.

Plus, large chain gyms pack members in by the dozens, and the program can be diminished by overcrowding or become uncomfortable. A good fitness company that offers quality group classes will likely charge anywhere from $60 – $130 per month, but again, it is worth the extra investment when compared to the environment and results.

Hiking, Walking, and Outdoors.

By far, my favorite form of exercise, and most cities provide access to parks, trails, and outdoor activities. There are dozens of options for the outdoor enthusiast or a person looking to add this component to their lifestyle. The cost of enjoying a long hike is negligible and aside from time and transportation, there is little cost associated with getting outside and exploring the beauty of our world.

Hikes and long walks can be enjoyed with partners, family, and pets, so plan some time outdoors and make a day of it. Camping is also another great way to get moving and can serve as a base for some longer day or destination hikes to get your body moving. While getting outdoors may seem overly simple, it is about creating a sustainable life change. In my experience, most people who connect with the outdoors this way stick to their nutrition and workout plans during the week, so they are ready for the weekend hike, boat trip, or hitting the mountainside.

Get Involved with Team or Individual Sports.

Organized team sports or adult leagues are a fantastic way to bring fun and focus to a workout program. Not only are some sports inherently active, but they all also require fitness training or conditioning. If you have a team sport you enjoy, most cities have dozens of leagues available for you to explore. Personally, I enjoy individual challenge sports like the difficult mud and obstacle runs or extended back-country kayaking, snowboarding, or mountaineering.

These passions fuel my fitness programs and keep me focused on more than just sets, reps, and meal planning. Again, your sport or physical activity should be woven into the fabric of your life to be more than just something you do. Because you are making a lifestyle change toward a fit body and strong discipline, adding these athletic options are all part of the structure that fortifies your resolve and results.

Remember, there is no silver bullet for fitness. Instead, it is a combination of components like the five items listed above and managing your food intake. Plain and simple, you must get your nutrition under control and ensure your energy expenditure and food consumption is appropriate for your goal. I hope you take these suggestions seriously and move your mindset to programs and activities that enhance the quality of your life and bring long-lasting health and wellness!

Chapter Seventeen

HOW TO CHOOSE A PERSONAL TRAINER OR COACH

In this chapter, we discuss live personal training and online coaching and training. They each have their advantages. With the power of the web, whenever you have a question, you connect online and search for resources on your given topic. But this can be a trap as there is so much information online, much of which is incorrect. A personal trainer or fitness coach may solve not just cost and time but can be a definitive resource for personalized answers to your fitness questions.

Live Personal Training Advantages

Programming

Decide on the kind of program you feel will bring the greatest level of personal commitment. On one side of the spectrum, some trainers specialize in militant forms of exercise or "boot camps" that push your body to the limit. On the other side, some trainers perform a full postural deviation assessment and scientifically design a custom program that will safely and effectively lead you to your goals through a progression. Your current condition level and goal will be a factor in choosing the kind of trainer you seek, so be objective about your ability and commitment.

Environment

Decide on the environment you feel would be the most motivating and attractive in which to train. Fitness venues range from classic box-chain gyms, private studios, industrial warehouse conversions, outdoor camps, or even at a residence. Remember, if you are not comfortable with your training environment, then it will be more challenging to focus on your personal trainer's guidance. Be sure the trainer and environment are a match to your needs.

Certification

Decide on a trainer with a nationally recognized fitness trainer certification. Ask about their education, certifications, and experience as it relates to your condition level and goal. It is recommended not to hire uncertified "trainers" or hobby fitness enthusiasts. Some of the most respected certification acronyms include NASM, ACSM, ACE, NESTA, NCSF, NETA, NFPT & NSCA. To be clear, certifications do not guarantee a trainer has personality or competence. Take your time and get to know the trainer in your first session and see that qualifications match charisma.

Cost Factors

Decide to pay for results. Remember, the price a trainer may charge is not always an indication of quality, but any trainer with experience and a successful track record will not be cheap. Expect to pay premiums for experienced and competent trainers and be glad for it. Nothing bitters the sweetness of a low price like poor service. On average, a half-hour session with a trainer will run around $35-$45 per session and most hour sessions range from $50-$100+ depending on the trainer or fitness club price structure. Most professional trainers will offer a free assessment session to give you a better idea of program design, trainer quality, and cost. Don't be cheap.

Communication

Communicate throughout the workout with your trainer. Feedback or adjustments are important, and this is usually a sign that your trainer is paying attention to how your body is responding to the program. Active communication throughout the session will only enhance your experience and rapport with the trainer.

Objective Measurements

Decide to continually assess your progress. A professional trainer is aware of the human ability to adapt to physical strain and will constantly be tweaking or changing your program to ensure your body progresses in stabilization, strength, and endurance. However, strive to be objective in your self-assessments and be honest about your nutrition, effort, and consistency. Working with a personal trainer is like a partnership and both parties must contribute to success.

Online Coaching and Training Advantages

We live in a world of packed schedules where convenience and speed can be the determining factor in our choices. Many of our convenient food options are caloric rich with poor nutritional density. Trying to balance exercise and reasonable food intake can be quite a challenge, so hiring an expert can make a huge difference in your wellness success.

Traditionally, you join a gym and hopefully hire a personal trainer and get the help of a professional. But not everyone can afford a private trainer or may simply not have time to schedule live sessions. However, technology is providing some outstanding new benefits that have made gaining information, education, and assistance in fitness even more accessible.

An online trainer is a fitness resource you can access without having to step outside your home. You do not have to visit the gym if you prefer home workouts, and you need not try and match schedules with a live trainer.

All communication is done through the internet or via a mobile app, and the best online coaches provide video or phone chats weekly or monthly. Once you choose an online coach, he or she can develop a custom exercise program for you and many offer nutrition services as well. On the internet, you can hire a coach no matter where they or you are located and is a cost-effective coaching solution in comparison to in-person-training.

Many online personal trainers also generally maintain a high level of interaction with their clients through emails, newsletters, videos, or webcams. If you find a trainer with poor communication, you can always find other highly qualified experts who will meet your expectations. Here are five reasons to consider online coaching:

Work out Anytime

Training at any time you want. Since you are not meeting with your personal trainer in person, you can complete your training at any time during the scheduled training days. This solves a common problem of having to choose time intervals that fit the busy schedules of you and your coach. Most online trainers will have your workouts built and loaded in a mobile app, so it's fun and convenient.

Work out Anywhere

Training where you want. When a training client uses an online personal trainer, he or she can train anywhere. Simply log in to your training account, check in for your workout, and begin your exercises. The best online trainers will have explanation videos for each exercise and include the number of sets, reps, and weight targets for most movements.

Affordability

According to the 2008 IDEA Personal Training Survey, the average price for personal training in the United States is $58 per hour. Unfortunately, most people cannot afford personal training for extended durations. However, at an estimated average of $100-$250 per month, most folks can afford online personal training, especially if they prioritize it like they do cable television or cell phones.

The real value of an online personal trainer is that he or she offers the same benefits of on-site personal training, one-on-one, but with significant cost savings. Yes, there are some disadvantages to online personal training, such as live form correction, on-the-spot encouragement, and appointment accountability. Yet many trainers have ways to overcome these challenges such as a webcam session, video submissions, or demonstrations.

Exceptional Value

Dollar for dollar, the benefits of an online personal trainer far outweigh the costs. You get all the expertise and tools for success you normally get with personal and in-person training.

If you choose the right coach, they will add value with custom workouts, meal plans, education, tips, motivation, and personalized connection. Many online trainers have a fair or excellent understanding of nutrition concepts as well.

Tip: Be careful of the online "coach" that uses templates or avoids communication! These are typically social media personalities and not professionals.

Avoid Gymtimidation

Some people are too self-conscious or ashamed to go to gyms or fitness centers. They fear being watched or intimidated by the fit crowd or feel they will look silly or lost.

Personal online training solves these problems by providing a higher level of privacy, allowing clients to work at their own pace and in their environmental comfort zone. Many online training clients work out exclusively from home and soon work their way to higher levels of self-confidence.

Chapter Eighteen
HOW TO CHOOSE A FITNESS FACILITY

Not all fitness centers are created equal, and not all gyms are right for everyone. The positive side of so much competition is the new variety of niche options available that provide more than just access to rows of equipment and focus on programming that improves the personal wellness and lifestyle of members and clients.

Generally, there are five fitness center or "gym" environments, and there is usually a difference in price, facility, amenities, staff, and even member base demographics. Here is a quick summary of each kind of club to help you choose the best fit for you and your wellness needs.

Corporate Chain Gyms & Franchises

Over the past twenty-five years, large corporate box-style fitness centers have spread across the United States. Many. One distinct advantage of joining this kind of gym is the accessibility to multiple locations and the consistency they can deliver in a facility, equipment, and group classes. The price of membership is typically affordable, and these clubs provide a range of cost options and membership terms.

As a veteran fitness professional, I must point out that corporate chain gyms have created a negative stereotype about sales, exercise, and even personal trainers. Corporate gyms survive on volume business and services are an afterthought to their model. In addition, they typically attract low-wage-earning employees and inexperienced personal trainers just entering their careers. Low price and high member traffic are also typical in many of the smaller franchise clubs, but operations can be hit or miss with franchisee-operated gyms.

The combination of hyper-focused sales and inexperienced staff can be repelling to a large portion of people looking for a total wellness program. However, many individuals gain benefits from having access to the wide variety of equipment and novelties available in the chain gym, and they can be a great resource for the avid exerciser or someone comfortable with the atmosphere of a traditional box gym. The popularity of this kind of environment has diminished in recent years as many consumers are seeking a more personalized and results-based program.

Boutique Personal Training Studios

Without question, working with the right certified personal trainer is a sure way to see significant results. Like many aspects of the fitness world, personal training has been devalued by big corporations driving down prices and hiring inferior trainers and pressuring a sales cycle. Not to say there are not some spectacular trainers working for corporate gyms, but most choose to leave the pressure cooker and open a studio or work for a company focused on real wellness services.

A professional personal trainer will create a specific program based on your condition level and ideal fitness objective. Good trainers will perform a comprehensive fitness assessment and develop a program to bring your body back into structural alignment and then progressively create interesting new workouts that safely and effectively deliver results. Provided you control your calorie intake.

The training environment can be diverse, so be sure the studio is comfortable for you and meets your needs. Some boutique training services can be done in your own home or the home of a trainer. However, serious professionals will have a studio facility or rent space from another fitness company. Like most specialized services, price is usually the biggest topic of concern for those interested in hiring a trainer.

However, the return on investment is often measured by improved flexibility, desired physique, endurance, strength, joint health, and cardiovascular fortitude. When seeking a personal trainer, price should not necessarily be the deciding factor. The studio environment is important, but you are hiring the trainer, so be sure you have a connection, and they are certified.

Working with the right personal trainer is by far the best way to achieve your results and will pay for itself over and over.

Olympic Style Gyms

Dozens of these warehouses and garage fitness centers are scattered through communities and have gained significant popularity over the past decade. These classes are designed to accommodate a smaller membership base and are known for intense workouts. Many maneuvers in these classes are based on Olympic-style liftings such as the snatch and clean and the jerk. In addition, these programs include high-volume repletion of deadlifts, squats, and overhead presses.

High-Intensity Interval Training is also woven into these classes to challenge your fitness. Unfortunately, many of these owner-operators are not certified trainers and the injury rate for this class type is notoriously high. I will also point out that many of the participants in these programs are not ready for this kind of workload and are already dispositioned for injury or excessive soreness.

Yet the attraction power comes from the sense of community these smaller gyms naturally create and the fact that you will no doubt be challenged by the routines. The price for this kind of fitness service can be greater than that of a corporate chain gym, but you get arguably more value for the dollar. Provided you have a competent coach or trainer ensuring safety and proper form.

The atmosphere can be gritty because of where most of the gyms are located. Warehouses, industrial spaces, or even home garages are common facility sites. This means they provide bare amenities if any, at all. If a locker room or even a water fountain is a necessity for you, this may not be the best fitness club option. However, some clubs in industrial areas have made a significant investment into the atmosphere, so it's best to check them out in person.

Yoga, Pilates, and Mind-Body Studios

The rising popularity of Yoga, Pilates, and other mind-body options are also the byproducts of consumers looking for alternatives to the corporate chain gym. However, these modalities also stand on their own merits. Typically, these fitness options are low-impact and can greatly reduce stress, increase flexibility, build core strength, and fortify joint stability.

Over the past decade, many studios have reduced some of the spiritual aspects and now focus more on the physiological component, but there is usually an option for either. Choosing the right studio is just as important as choosing the right gym. Each location has its ambiance, culture, and instructor quality.

Enjoying a two or three-day trial may be beneficial, so take a few classes and decide which instructor and time work best for you. Price can range from medium to high, but most of these studios are specialized and charge accordingly. You get what you pay for, so if you like the program and people, the price should be the least of your concerns. It's only expensive if you don't attend classes.

Luxury Brand or Country Clubs

Luxury brand clubs can be a corporate chain, small multi-club group, or single location entity. Most of these clubs have high-level amenities such as racquet sports, swimming pools, recreational water features, bars, restaurants, and opulent locker rooms. Some of the pricey options have an onsite salon & spa and even some medical offices. While many of these luxuries are not necessary to achieve fitness results, they can enhance your experience or even motivate you to work out more consistently.

There can be a heavy social aspect to this kind of club, but that is true in nearly all fitness options. Yet for all the glamor, the machines are the same as the cheap corporate volume gym across the street and the dumbbells all weigh the same. In a sense, joining a luxury club is more for exclusivity, social connection, and ambiance than it is for fitness. Prices can be very high compared to other options, but some people find the extra cost worth it as the amenities are unrivaled and the staff is typically more customer service savvy.

Remember, the purpose of joining a fitness center or enrolling in a service is to achieve your fitness goals. While I typically lean toward live personal training studios and the luxury health club, I encourage you to get involved in the program that will deliver results and keep you interested in making your wellness a lifestyle and daily priority!

Chapter Nineteen
HOW TO OVERCOME HOLIDAY FOOD TEMPTATIONS

The holidays are a special time to share with friends and family, yet so many people struggle with maintaining a healthy lifestyle during the season. Excessive food consumption, lack of activity, party commitments, travel, and other stresses can take control and before you know it, you have gained some unwanted body fat or feel overwhelmed with obligations or the looming reality of the holiday season aftermath. Here are 5 simple healthy holiday eating tips to survive the holiday food temptation:

Set A Personal Calorie Limit

Each day or before every party, commit to a limit on calorie consumption. Take a moment to consider your favorite dishes, treats, or traditional foods and get some information on approximate calorie values. This research will take very little time and there are dozens of great resources online that explain the approximate calorie value of most foods.

Decide how much you are willing to consume, understanding that moderation is key. It's perfectly normal and healthy to indulge occasionally during the holiday, so don't let the concept of overeating control your mood or outlook. Simply make a plan and stick to it as close as possible.

You will feel the satisfaction of maintaining your commitment while limiting the days you overconsume. This will make the holiday far more enjoyable, and you will have far less work to do on your figure when the season ends.

Choose Only Your Favorite Foods

Now that you have a calorie goal, be picky about what you consume and make it count. It's the holidays, and they are supposed to be a time of celebration and communion. Pick foods traditional to you or something you look forward to each season.

Pass up the store-bought goods and reconsider that handful of generic candy. Instead, enjoy a modest piece of grandma's epic homemade pie or your cousin's legendary scratch fudge. When it comes to the big dinner, go lite on the servings, and have a modest portion of all your favorites.

A great way to lower the calorie load is to go easy on the mound of starches such as mashed potatoes and stuffing surrounded by an ocean of gravy or cut the pie serving in half. Remember, moderation is key, and you truly can balance reasonable food intake while still enjoying the holiday.

Keep Active

One of the most important health decisions you can make year-round is to remain active. The holidays often pose a challenge because our schedules are usually altered, and social calendars can be packed. However, it is very possible to remain active to a large degree, no matter how full your week looks.

Some useful ways to keep yourself active include attending a regularly scheduled fitness class, hire a personal trainer so you have an appointment, or commit to a morning or afternoon walk on your own or with the family. Maintaining at least a half-hour or better yet, an hour of activity each day will improve your mood, reduce stress, and help balance the added calories you may be consuming.

Manage Your Alcohol Consumption

Many people enjoy the season with traditional cocktails or Champaign toasts. Again, moderation is key, so just remember a few facts. Alcohol contains seven calories per gram, and it can add up quickly. Two glasses of sparkling wine can exceed 240 calories and two martinis can top 200 calories.

A mug of spiked cider can even get up to 300 calories in some recipes. Aside from the nutritional side, alcohol also inhibits the release of glucose, and this can alter blood sugar levels and metabolic rate.

Plus, alcohol is a powerful agent in judgment impairment. Aside from the crude joke you tell at dinner, much to the horror of your mother, you may be more likely to forget your calorie goal or absentmindedly overindulge.

Commit to a Lifelong Wellness Plan

Without question, coming into a holiday season with a defined, scheduled, and committed plan already in place makes a huge difference. Those who commit to their wellbeing often come through the holiday mostly unscathed and are right back into their normal fitness routines once the season ends. One-time resolutions are useless, as I'm sure you already know from your own experience.

Success in health and fitness comes from a year-long personal commitment and positive habits. Wellness is a personal responsibility and acting early and keeping momentum through all of life's seasons makes navigating the holiday stress-free and rewarding. Don't let the bounty of the year or the holiday season be stressful. Follow the 5 steps above and stop the cycle!

Chapter Twenty
HOW TO STAY ON TRACK WHEN TRAVELING

Many people struggle to maintain adherence to fitness and nutrition schedules while traveling. This is true for vacation and business travel. While each travel type presents its unique challenges, we will explore several tips for staying on track with proper food management and prioritizing exercise.

Commit Unconditionally to Your Plan

This may sound obvious, but if you do not decide to fully commit and plan your fitness and consumption into your workout plans, then you will likely struggle even more when traveling. Contemplation is only part of the equation. You must act by considering your travel schedule, the distance between meals, availability of space or fitness center on the road, food availability, and the quality of food sources.

I also recommend you look at your travel schedule and add workouts into spaces or places most likely to accommodate the need and mentally resolve to make it happen. The commitment concept of fitness & nutrition planning for travel is true for vacation, holiday celebrations, or business.

Prepare Snacks for Transit Time

This is a simple strategy to avoid missing meals or making a poor food choice. By planning your schedule and packing some travel-friendly snacks, you can ensure you are not in a situation where you get overly hungry, lose energy, or consume something that you would not otherwise choose to eat. Plus, the selection may not be ideal or in line with your regular nutrition plan. Aside from not being miserably hungry on a trip, another benefit to snack planning is you maintain full control of your nutrition. I suggest you pre-plan snacks and separate portions according to your needs and travel situation. Instead of bringing a whole warehouse club jug of nuts, simply potion out your ration and put it into a baggie or small meal storage container.

This will also help you avoid over-snacking. Some excellent travel snacks include portioned nuts, fresh or dried fruits, raw veggies, boiled eggs, jerky, and whole-food snack bars. You can also prepare smoothies or protein shakes ahead of time and keep them in your cooler if travel accommodations allow.

Research Destination Meal and Fitness Options

Whenever possible, research your waypoints and destination to see what the food scene looks like or if there is a fitness center available. I always do an online search and investigate all the food options around my travel spots or where I know I will stop or stay. This is easy if you are on a train or in a car and makes the trip a little more fun knowing the layout of some destinations.

I do the same thing for fitness centers as well. Most hotels have a modest gym, but more often than not, they are pretty pathetic. The good news is there are over two hundred thousand fitness centers worldwide, you will probably have an option beyond the hotel. Nearly all gyms allow single day use for a nominal fee and I always find it fascinating and fun to explore different gyms across the world and stay on track with my workouts.

Prioritize Some Form of Daily Exercise

I suggest you prioritize your workouts and schedule them like you would any other travel event. Even if there is not a fitness center available, you can and should plan a short body-weight workout. Many of my clients travel with resistance bands or I send them follow-along workout videos they can do right in their hotel room with minimal space.

I also recommend you try and keep workouts close to your normal schedule when you can to increase the likelihood of adherence. Prioritizing your fitness comes back to a commitment to your momentum and I have never had anyone tell me they regret keeping discipline and staying on their plan when traveling.

Remain Hydrated and Well Rested

Travel can be a special kind of exhausting, and it is easy to neglect hydration and rest. Whenever possible, carry water with you so it's always accessible and plan for rest times. This is especially true for air travel because of air humidity, dryness, and pressurization. Dehydration and lack of rest can interfere with the enjoyment of travel and make working out even more difficult and daunting. Low energy is a fast track to skipping workouts, and you need every advantage when you travel to keep to your plan.

Balance Indulgence with Moderation

Whether your travel is for business or pleasure, balancing indulgence with moderation is highly recommended. If you are traveling for business and going to a cocktail reception with clients, then simply plan for this and have already completed your workout in the morning and choose lower-calorie cocktails. Wine, beer, and low or no-sugar drinks are ideal. If you are on vacation, then day drinking, or some overeating is just fine if you moderate.

Make sure you have adjusted your workouts to balance this and avoid consecutive days of overindulgence. We often spend so much time preparing our physique for a vacation and then come back to reality and then have to repair the damage. Instead, I recommend a nice healthy balance to enjoy aspects that make vacations so enjoyable.

People are occasionally surprised by my philosophy on sustainable lifestyles and applying moderation to enhance the quality of an experience but still maintain control. This means I do not subscribe to the popular mainstream media, personal trainer, or nutrition coach approach of promoting deprivation, guilting people, or creating absolute restriction.

Fitness and nutrition should be sustainable and there is room for moderation on special occasions. If you follow these 6 steps, then you will be managing your fitness and nutrition lifestyle, which I hail as a success. Further, managing this lifestyle while traveling is just part of the process and your fitness success doesn't pause when you travel, you must take it with you.

Chapter Twenty-One
HOW TO KEEP YOUR RESOLUTIONS

I rarely advocate for resolutions, yet I discuss it here because so many people do. I feel it is such a common cultural and social normality that it is worth discussing. However, there is no substitution for making systemic personal change through deliberate habit alteration. Anyhow, the same thing happens year after year. Millions of people around the world make New Year resolutions such as:

- I want to lose weight
- I want to find and enjoy a lasting relationship
- I want to stop smoking or drinking
- I want to change my habits

But one month into the New Year, and already a lot of individuals have faltered and deviated from their resolutions.

Why Resolutions Fail

Most New Year resolutions fail because people make their goals unrealistic and lose the motivation to attain them. In fitness and nutrition resolutions, failure is related to several factors, including lack of true desire to change, failure to alter root cause habits, and choosing a fad or gimmick instead of a sustainable solution. Another huge issue for most folks is fear of the gym and lack of fitness knowledge.

Also, many people find that fitness and nutrition are much more difficult than they were expecting and did not get the results, no matter how unrealistic, they were hoping for. Taking it one step at a time and setting yourself up for success before the New Year arrives is the key. But why wait until the next year when you can start right now? Here are five tips to consider any time of the year:

Be Specific and Realistic

Most people, at the onset of the New Year, look for a quick fix or go all-in on the latest fad or gimmick. Sadly, we set our goals outside of reasonable and fail to create a strong plan to manage our food intake, work out on a schedule and eliminate influences in our lives contrary to our goals. Instead, pick a few goals or just one at a time that is not too difficult to attain.

Try improving your plank hold, increase your ability to do push-ups, or get to the gym at least thirty minutes every other day. Take some time to educate yourself on reasonable expectations for results and resolve to work hard even when those results are slow to come. Fitness is cumulative and increases in interest, just like a good savings account. You must keep putting in the effort to see it grow.

Set A Schedule

If you fail to plan, you plan to fail. Define a monthly schedule of workout commitments along with the duration, exercise type, and frequency. We will be more likely to follow a well-balanced plan instead of just taking random classes or undefined cardio. Achieving a weight loss goal within six months is reasonable; participating in a professionally guided training program for three months is also realistic and so on.

Expecting to lose several pounds of fat within days is nonsensical. Create a schedule that involves taking steps daily or weekly and have some loose benchmarks in place so you can affirm progress. Do not be discouraged by slow results. This may indicate you have adapted to your workouts, and you can get out of that rut with some alterations and changes to intensity. Refer to your schedule and update the plan as you go.

Work Toward Progress, Not Perfection

Exercise takes practice and developing strength, endurance, and ultimately, fat loss takes time. Look for little signs of progress each day and do not look for perfection at the expense of progress. Ensure your planned outcomes are not based on external projections as we all have different shapes, genetic gifts, and separate body types. Specify goals that are not only related to your aesthetics but also can be measured in other ways. Increasing your deadlift, doing a pull-up, or lifting your heavy, aging dog into the car are great functional goals.

Start Practicing Positive Affirmations

If you think you cannot stick with something, you are right. If you think you can, then you can. We all need to improve our internal conversations and practice treating ourselves with courtesy and respect. Banish negative thoughts about yourself or "hating" parts of your body. Instead, embrace your situation and work hard to change it. Don't be a bully and tear yourself down. Build internal trust with yourself by maintaining your commitment and affirming your value daily. Say positive things to yourself, such as:

- I will not allow myself or anyone else to detour me with words or actions.
- I will treat myself with love and care.
- I will do this with a joyful spirit.
- I will reach my intended goal.

These positive affirmations will help you to stay on track but, moreover, will alter your perspective from negative to positive.

Change Your Habits, Change Your Life

A problem with most resolutions is that they ignore the root cause, which is your bad habits. To make long-term change, you must create specific strategies to help yourself overcome food temptation triggers, set realistic goals, establish rewards, identify obstacles, and attain the mindset for long-term success. Work hard to replace those negative habits with positive behaviors that are sustainable.

ADDITIONAL RESOURCES

In this section, I have included several powerful resources to help you organize your weeks, get inspired with meal plans, and outline some basic types of workouts with an example of each.

90-Day Habit Weekly Success Journal

I hope that this tool provides you with a visual reminder and tactile way to track your workouts, nutrition, and new healthy lifestyle habits. Here is a brief overview of how to use this journal:

Each page represents a week with 7 total days where you can make a quick mark about your efforts with a simple check box.

• The standard daily tasks are "Workout Completed" and "Food Intake Logged" but there are two blank spaces for you to list some of your personal goals each day.

• It is recommended that at the beginning of each week, you write in a personal goal or two on each day, so you have a strong personal focus on short-term weekly success.

• Use the N/A box only if that day was not a scheduled workout day.

• Nutrition should be logged or at least intuitively managed to ensure proper intake of energy and food quality.

• Because you set your personal goals in the two blank lines, either you achieved that goal, or you did not.

• The last worksheet has an empty circle for a new week for you to fill in so you can continue your journaling.

Here are some personal daily goal ideas:

I will not eat added sugar	I will add 20 minutes to cardio
I will not drink sodas	I will try for a new Personal Best
I will not drink alcohol	I will compliment myself
I will not exceed my calories	I will not eat fast food
I will not skip stretching	I will not make excuses

SUCCESS JOURNAL // WEEK ①

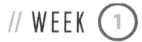

DATE _____

MONDAY	YES // NO // N/A
Workout Completed:	☐ ☐ ☐
Food Intake Logged:	☐ ☐
	☐ ☐
	☐ ☐

TUESDAY	YES // NO // N/A
Workout Completed:	☐ ☐ ☐
Food Intake Logged:	☐ ☐
	☐ ☐
	☐ ☐

WEDNESDAY	YES // NO // N/A
Workout Completed:	☐ ☐ ☐
Food Intake Logged:	☐ ☐
	☐ ☐
	☐ ☐

THURSDAY	YES // NO // N/A
Workout Completed:	☐ ☐ ☐
Food Intake Logged:	☐ ☐
	☐ ☐
	☐ ☐

FRIDAY	YES // NO // N/A
Workout Completed:	☐ ☐ ☐
Food Intake Logged:	☐ ☐
	☐ ☐
	☐ ☐

SATURDAY	YES // NO // N/A
Workout Completed:	☐ ☐ ☐
Food Intake Logged:	☐ ☐
	☐ ☐
	☐ ☐

SUNDAY	YES // NO // N/A
Workout Completed:	☐ ☐ ☐
Food Intake Logged:	☐ ☐
	☐ ☐
	☐ ☐

WEEKLY NOTES:

SUCCESS JOURNAL

// WEEK ②

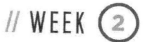

DATE _____

MONDAY | YES // NO // N/A
Workout Completed: ☐ ☐ ☐
Food Intake Logged: ☐ ☐
☐ ☐
☐ ☐

TUESDAY | YES // NO // N/A
Workout Completed: ☐ ☐ ☐
Food Intake Logged: ☐ ☐
☐ ☐
☐ ☐

WEDNESDAY | YES // NO // N/A
Workout Completed: ☐ ☐ ☐
Food Intake Logged: ☐ ☐
☐ ☐
☐ ☐

THURSDAY | YES // NO // N/A
Workout Completed: ☐ ☐ ☐
Food Intake Logged: ☐ ☐
☐ ☐
☐ ☐

FRIDAY | YES // NO // N/A
Workout Completed: ☐ ☐ ☐
Food Intake Logged: ☐ ☐
☐ ☐
☐ ☐

SATURDAY | YES // NO // N/A
Workout Completed: ☐ ☐ ☐
Food Intake Logged: ☐ ☐
☐ ☐
☐ ☐

SUNDAY | YES // NO // N/A
Workout Completed: ☐ ☐ ☐
Food Intake Logged: ☐ ☐
☐ ☐
☐ ☐

WEEKLY NOTES:
_____
_____
_____
_____

SUCCESS JOURNAL // WEEK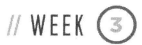

DATE _____

MONDAY	YES // NO // N/A
Workout Completed:	☐ ☐ ☐
Food Intake Logged:	☐ ☐
	☐ ☐
	☐ ☐

TUESDAY	YES // NO // N/A
Workout Completed:	☐ ☐ ☐
Food Intake Logged:	☐ ☐
	☐ ☐
	☐ ☐

WEDNESDAY	YES // NO // N/A
Workout Completed:	☐ ☐ ☐
Food Intake Logged:	☐ ☐
	☐ ☐
	☐ ☐

THURSDAY	YES // NO // N/A
Workout Completed:	☐ ☐ ☐
Food Intake Logged:	☐ ☐
	☐ ☐
	☐ ☐

FRIDAY	YES // NO // N/A
Workout Completed:	☐ ☐ ☐
Food Intake Logged:	☐ ☐
	☐ ☐
	☐ ☐

SATURDAY	YES // NO // N/A
Workout Completed:	☐ ☐ ☐
Food Intake Logged:	☐ ☐
	☐ ☐
	☐ ☐

SUNDAY	YES // NO // N/A
Workout Completed:	☐ ☐ ☐
Food Intake Logged:	☐ ☐
	☐ ☐
	☐ ☐

WEEKLY NOTES

SUCCESS JOURNAL // WEEK ④

DATE _____

MONDAY	YES // NO // N/A
Workout Completed:	☐ ☐ ☐
Food Intake Logged:	☐ ☐
	☐ ☐
	☐ ☐

TUESDAY	YES // NO // N/A
Workout Completed:	☐ ☐ ☐
Food Intake Logged:	☐ ☐
	☐ ☐
	☐ ☐

WEDNESDAY	YES // NO // N/A
Workout Completed:	☐ ☐ ☐
Food Intake Logged:	☐ ☐
	☐ ☐
	☐ ☐

THURSDAY	YES // NO // N/A
Workout Completed:	☐ ☐ ☐
Food Intake Logged:	☐ ☐
	☐ ☐
	☐ ☐

FRIDAY	YES // NO // N/A
Workout Completed:	☐ ☐ ☐
Food Intake Logged:	☐ ☐
	☐ ☐
	☐ ☐

SATURDAY	YES // NO // N/A
Workout Completed:	☐ ☐ ☐
Food Intake Logged:	☐ ☐
	☐ ☐
	☐ ☐

SUNDAY	YES // NO // N/A
Workout Completed:	☐ ☐ ☐
Food Intake Logged:	☐ ☐
	☐ ☐
	☐ ☐

WEEKLY NOTES:

SUCCESS JOURNAL

// WEEK ⑤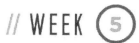

DATE _____

MONDAY	YES // NO // N/A
Workout Completed:	☐ ☐ ☐
Food Intake Logged:	☐ ☐
	☐ ☐
	☐ ☐

TUESDAY	YES // NO // N/A
Workout Completed:	☐ ☐ ☐
Food Intake Logged:	☐ ☐
	☐ ☐
	☐ ☐

WEDNESDAY	YES // NO // N/A
Workout Completed:	☐ ☐ ☐
Food Intake Logged:	☐ ☐
	☐ ☐
	☐ ☐

THURSDAY	YES // NO // N/A
Workout Completed:	☐ ☐ ☐
Food Intake Logged:	☐ ☐
	☐ ☐
	☐ ☐

FRIDAY	YES // NO // N/A
Workout Completed:	☐ ☐ ☐
Food Intake Logged:	☐ ☐
	☐ ☐
	☐ ☐

SATURDAY	YES // NO // N/A
Workout Completed:	☐ ☐ ☐
Food Intake Logged:	☐ ☐
	☐ ☐
	☐ ☐

SUNDAY	YES // NO // N/A
Workout Completed:	☐ ☐ ☐
Food Intake Logged:	☐ ☐
	☐ ☐
	☐ ☐

WEEKLY NOTES:

SUCCESS JOURNAL // WEEK 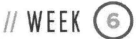 6

DATE _____

MONDAY	YES // NO // N/A
Workout Completed:	☐ ☐ ☐
Food Intake Logged:	☐ ☐
	☐ ☐
	☐ ☐

TUESDAY	YES // NO // N/A
Workout Completed:	☐ ☐ ☐
Food Intake Logged:	☐ ☐
	☐ ☐
	☐ ☐

WEDNESDAY	YES // NO // N/A
Workout Completed:	☐ ☐ ☐
Food Intake Logged:	☐ ☐
	☐ ☐
	☐ ☐

THURSDAY	YES // NO // N/A
Workout Completed:	☐ ☐ ☐
Food Intake Logged:	☐ ☐
	☐ ☐
	☐ ☐

FRIDAY	YES // NO // N/A
Workout Completed:	☐ ☐ ☐
Food Intake Logged:	☐ ☐
	☐ ☐
	☐ ☐

SATURDAY	YES // NO // N/A
Workout Completed:	☐ ☐ ☐
Food Intake Logged:	☐ ☐
	☐ ☐
	☐ ☐

SUNDAY	YES // NO // N/A
Workout Completed:	☐ ☐ ☐
Food Intake Logged:	☐ ☐
	☐ ☐
	☐ ☐

WEEKLY NOTES:

SUCCESS JOURNAL

// WEEK ⑦

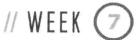

DATE _____

MONDAY	YES // NO // N/A
Workout Completed:	☐ ☐ ☐
Food Intake Logged:	☐ ☐
	☐ ☐
	☐ ☐

TUESDAY	YES // NO // N/A
Workout Completed:	☐ ☐ ☐
Food Intake Logged:	☐ ☐
	☐ ☐
	☐ ☐

WEDNESDAY	YES // NO // N/A
Workout Completed:	☐ ☐ ☐
Food Intake Logged:	☐ ☐
	☐ ☐
	☐ ☐

THURSDAY	YES // NO // N/A
Workout Completed:	☐ ☐ ☐
Food Intake Logged:	☐ ☐
	☐ ☐
	☐ ☐

FRIDAY	YES // NO // N/A
Workout Completed:	☐ ☐ ☐
Food Intake Logged:	☐ ☐
	☐ ☐
	☐ ☐

SATURDAY	YES // NO // N/A
Workout Completed:	☐ ☐ ☐
Food Intake Logged:	☐ ☐
	☐ ☐
	☐ ☐

SUNDAY	YES // NO // N/A
Workout Completed:	☐ ☐ ☐
Food Intake Logged:	☐ ☐
	☐ ☐
	☐ ☐

WEEKLY NOTES:

SUCCESS JOURNAL

// WEEK 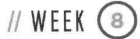 (8)

DATE _____

MONDAY	YES // NO // N/A
Workout Completed:	☐ ☐ ☐
Food Intake Logged:	☐ ☐
	☐ ☐
	☐ ☐

TUESDAY	YES // NO // N/A
Workout Completed:	☐ ☐ ☐
Food Intake Logged:	☐ ☐
	☐ ☐
	☐ ☐

WEDNESDAY	YES // NO // N/A
Workout Completed:	☐ ☐ ☐
Food Intake Logged:	☐ ☐
	☐ ☐
	☐ ☐

THURSDAY	YES // NO // N/A
Workout Completed:	☐ ☐ ☐
Food Intake Logged:	☐ ☐
	☐ ☐
	☐ ☐

FRIDAY	YES // NO // N/A
Workout Completed:	☐ ☐ ☐
Food Intake Logged:	☐ ☐
	☐ ☐
	☐ ☐

SATURDAY	YES // NO // N/A
Workout Completed:	☐ ☐ ☐
Food Intake Logged:	☐ ☐
	☐ ☐
	☐ ☐

SUNDAY	YES // NO // N/A
Workout Completed:	☐ ☐ ☐
Food Intake Logged:	☐ ☐
	☐ ☐
	☐ ☐

WEEKLY NOTES:

SUCCESS JOURNAL

// WEEK ⑨

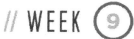

DATE _____

MONDAY	YES // NO // N/A
Workout Completed:	☐ ☐ ☐
Food Intake Logged:	☐ ☐
	☐ ☐
	☐ ☐

TUESDAY	YES // NO // N/A
Workout Completed:	☐ ☐ ☐
Food Intake Logged:	☐ ☐
	☐ ☐
	☐ ☐

WEDNESDAY	YES // NO // N/A
Workout Completed:	☐ ☐ ☐
Food Intake Logged:	☐ ☐
	☐ ☐
	☐ ☐

THURSDAY	YES // NO // N/A
Workout Completed:	☐ ☐ ☐
Food Intake Logged:	☐ ☐
	☐ ☐
	☐ ☐

FRIDAY	YES // NO // N/A
Workout Completed:	☐ ☐ ☐
Food Intake Logged:	☐ ☐
	☐ ☐
	☐ ☐

SATURDAY	YES // NO // N/A
Workout Completed:	☐ ☐ ☐
Food Intake Logged:	☐ ☐
	☐ ☐
	☐ ☐

SUNDAY	YES // NO // N/A
Workout Completed:	☐ ☐ ☐
Food Intake Logged:	☐ ☐
	☐ ☐
	☐ ☐

WEEKLY NOTES:

SUCCESS JOURNAL

// WEEK 10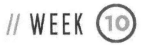

DATE _____

MONDAY

	YES // NO // N/A		
Workout Completed:	☐	☐	☐
Food Intake Logged:	☐	☐	
	☐	☐	
	☐	☐	

TUESDAY

	YES // NO // N/A		
Workout Completed:	☐	☐	☐
Food Intake Logged:	☐	☐	
	☐	☐	
	☐	☐	

WEDNESDAY

	YES // NO // N/A		
Workout Completed:	☐	☐	☐
Food Intake Logged:	☐	☐	
	☐	☐	
	☐	☐	

THURSDAY

	YES // NO // N/A		
Workout Completed:	☐	☐	☐
Food Intake Logged:	☐	☐	
	☐	☐	
	☐	☐	

FRIDAY

	YES // NO // N/A		
Workout Completed:	☐	☐	☐
Food Intake Logged:	☐	☐	
	☐	☐	
	☐	☐	

SATURDAY

	YES // NO // N/A		
Workout Completed:	☐	☐	☐
Food Intake Logged:	☐	☐	
	☐	☐	
	☐	☐	

SUNDAY

	YES // NO // N/A		
Workout Completed:	☐	☐	☐
Food Intake Logged:	☐	☐	
	☐	☐	
	☐	☐	

WEEKLY NOTES:

_____
_____
_____
_____

SUCCESS JOURNAL

// WEEK (11)

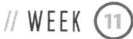

DATE _____

MONDAY	YES // NO // N/A
Workout Completed:	☐ ☐ ☐
Food Intake Logged:	☐ ☐
	☐ ☐
	☐ ☐

TUESDAY	YES // NO // N/A
Workout Completed:	☐ ☐ ☐
Food Intake Logged:	☐ ☐
	☐ ☐
	☐ ☐

WEDNESDAY	YES // NO // N/A
Workout Completed:	☐ ☐ ☐
Food Intake Logged:	☐ ☐
	☐ ☐
	☐ ☐

THURSDAY	YES // NO // N/A
Workout Completed:	☐ ☐ ☐
Food Intake Logged:	☐ ☐
	☐ ☐
	☐ ☐

FRIDAY	YES // NO // N/A
Workout Completed:	☐ ☐ ☐
Food Intake Logged:	☐ ☐
	☐ ☐
	☐ ☐

SATURDAY	YES // NO // N/A
Workout Completed:	☐ ☐ ☐
Food Intake Logged:	☐ ☐
	☐ ☐
	☐ ☐

SUNDAY	YES // NO // N/A
Workout Completed:	☐ ☐ ☐
Food Intake Logged:	☐ ☐
	☐ ☐
	☐ ☐

WEEKLY NOTES:

SUCCESS JOURNAL

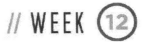

// WEEK (12)

DATE _____

MONDAY	YES // NO // N/A
Workout Completed:	☐ ☐ ☐
Food Intake Logged:	☐ ☐
	☐ ☐
	☐ ☐

TUESDAY	YES // NO // N/A
Workout Completed:	☐ ☐ ☐
Food Intake Logged:	☐ ☐
	☐ ☐
	☐ ☐

WEDNESDAY	YES // NO // N/A
Workout Completed:	☐ ☐ ☐
Food Intake Logged:	☐ ☐
	☐ ☐
	☐ ☐

THURSDAY	YES // NO // N/A
Workout Completed:	☐ ☐ ☐
Food Intake Logged:	☐ ☐
	☐ ☐
	☐ ☐

FRIDAY	YES // NO // N/A
Workout Completed:	☐ ☐ ☐
Food Intake Logged:	☐ ☐
	☐ ☐
	☐ ☐

SATURDAY	YES // NO // N/A
Workout Completed:	☐ ☐ ☐
Food Intake Logged:	☐ ☐
	☐ ☐
	☐ ☐

SUNDAY	YES // NO // N/A
Workout Completed:	☐ ☐ ☐
Food Intake Logged:	☐ ☐
	☐ ☐
	☐ ☐

WEEKLY NOTES:

COMPREHENSIVE MEAL PLANS

I have included a set of meal plans ranging from 1,200 calories, 1,600 calories, 2,000 calories, and 2,400 calories. These plans include seven days of balanced, nutrient-dense meals designed to serve as a baseline in your meal planning. At the end of the meal plan section, I have included a Food Exchange List. This is a tool used to swap foods out and maintain relative calorie intake aligned with your targets yet assist you with adding variety.

Keep in mind, it is important to first consider your overall activity and structured exercise to determine your potential caloric expenditure. Once you have an estimated daily output, you can then structure a nutritious meal plan to accommodate your daily need and desired results.

If you need help choosing a calorie range, review the previous chapter "Where to Start with Nutrition" and learn how to estimate your calorie needs by calculating your Basal Metabolic Rate (BMR) and Total Daily Energy Expenditure (TDEE) as it relates to your goals.

1,200 CALORIE MEAL PLAN OUTLINES

1200 CALORIE MEAL PLAN

DAY 1

Breakfast
7:00 AM

drinking water	2 Cup(s)	0 cal
whole eggs, scrambled	2 large	182 cal
whole grain rolled oats, dry	1/3 Cup(s)	100 cal
raisins, seedless	1/4 cup	123 cal

MEAL TOTAL: Calories 405 cal / Carbs 53 g (52%) / Protein 13 g (13%) / Fat 16 g (35%) / Fluid 1

Snack
10:00 AM

smooth peanut butter, no salt	1 Tbsp	94 cal
apples	1/2 small	28 cal
drinking water	2 Cup(s)	0 cal
cottage cheese, non-fat	3/4 Cup(s)	78 cal

MEAL TOTAL: Calories 200 cal / Carbs 18 g (34%) / Protein 15 g (30%) / Fat 8 g (36%) / Fluid 21

Lunch
12:00 PM

drinking water	2 Cup(s)	0 cal
whole wheat tortillas	1/2 tortilla	64 cal
turkey breast, roasted	5 oz	193 cal
romaine lettuce	2 leaf	2 cal
hummus, lower sodium	1 Tbsp	26 cal

MEAL TOTAL: Calories 285 cal / Carbs 12 g (17%) / Protein 45 g (63%) / Fat 6 g (20%) / Fluid 20

Dinner
6:00 PM

cauliflower, no salt, boiled	1 Cup(s)	29 cal
yellowfin tuna fish, cooked	3 oz	111 cal
wild rice, cooked	1/2 Cup(s)	83 cal
lentil beans, no salt, boiled	1/3 Cup(s)	77 cal
extra virgin olive oil	1/2 tsp	20 cal
drinking water	2 Cup(s)	0 cal

MEAL TOTAL: Calories 318 cal / Carbs 36 g (44%) / Protein 36 g (45%) / Fat 4 g (11%) / Fluid 25

DAY 1 TOTAL: Calories 1,208 cal / **Carbs** 119 g (39%) / **Protein** 110 g (36%) / **Fat** 34 g (25%) / **Fluid** 8

1200 CALORIE MEAL PLAN

DAY 2			

Breakfast
7:00 AM

drinking water	1 Cup(s)	0 cal
skim milk with calcium	1 1/2 Cup(s)	130 cal
multi-grain cheerios cereal	1/2 Cup(s)	60 cal
whole eggs, scrambled	1 large	91 cal
egg whites, cooked	4 large	69 cal

MEAL TOTAL: Calories 349 cal / **Carbs** 32 g (38%) / **Protein** 34 g (41%) / **Fat** 8 g (21%) / **Fluid** 25

Snack
10:00 AM

drinking water	2 Cup(s)	0 cal
cashews	1 oz	157 cal
oranges	1 fruit	69 cal

MEAL TOTAL: Calories 225 cal / **Carbs** 26 g (43%) / **Protein** 6 g (11%) / **Fat** 13 g (46%) / **Fluid** 20

Lunch
12:00 PM

olive oil, mayonnaise, light	1 tsp	16 cal
iced tea, green	16 fl oz	0 cal
tomatoes	1/4 Cup(s)	8 cal
avocados	1/4 cup	58 cal
chicken, boneless, roasted	3 oz	142 cal
whole-wheat pita bread	1 small	74 cal

MEAL TOTAL: Calories 299 cal / **Carbs** 21 g (27%) / **Protein** 25 g (33%) / **Fat** 13 g (40%) / **Fluid** 21

Dinner
6:00 PM

green snap beans, no salt, boiled	1 Cup(s)	44 cal
yams, no salt, boiled or baked	1 1/2 Cup(s)	237 cal
drinking water	2 Cup(s)	0 cal
beef t-bone, broiled	3 oz	161 cal

MEAL TOTAL: Calories 441 cal / **Carbs** 66 g (59%) / **Protein** 28 g (25%) / **Fat** 8 g (16%) / **Fluid** 26

DAY 2 TOTAL: Calories 1,315 cal / **Carbs** 145 g (43%) / **Protein** 93 g (28%) / **Fat** 42 g (29%) / **Fluid** 92

1200 CALORIE MEAL PLAN

DAY 3

Breakfast
7:00 AM

smooth peanut butter, no salt	1 1/2 Tbsp	141 cal
skim milk with calcium	1 1/2 Cup(s)	130 cal
drinking water	1 Cup(s)	0 cal
whole wheat mini bagel	1/2 bagel	50 cal

MEAL TOTAL: Calories 321 cal / **Carbs** 33 g (40%) / **Protein** 21 g (25%) / **Fat** 13 g (35%) / **Fluid** 1

Snack
10:00 AM

bananas	1 small	90 cal
drinking water	2 Cup(s)	0 cal
nut and raisin granola bars	1/2 bar	64 cal

MEAL TOTAL: Calories 153 cal / **Carbs** 32 g (78%) / **Protein** 2 g (5%) / **Fat** 3 g (17%) / **Fluid** 19

Lunch
12:00 PM

drinking water	2 Cup(s)	0 cal
tuna fish, very low-sodium, in water	8 oz	224 cal
romaine lettuce	2 leaf	2 cal
olive oil, mayonnaise, light	1 tsp	16 cal
whole wheat tortillas	1 tortilla	127 cal

MEAL TOTAL: Calories 369 cal / **Carbs** 20 g (21%) / **Protein** 55 g (58%) / **Fat** 9 g (21%) / **Fluid** 17

Dinner
6:00 PM

marinara spaghetti sauce, ready to serve	1/4 Cup(s)	31 cal
green snap beans, no salt, boiled	1 1/2 Cup(s)	66 cal
drinking water	2 Cup(s)	0 cal
italian spiced pork chops	1 serving	100 cal
rice penne pasta, low-carb	1 oz	104 cal

MEAL TOTAL: Calories 300 cal / **Carbs** 44 g (57%) / **Protein** 24 g (32%) / **Fat** 4 g (11%) / **Fluid** 26

DAY 3 TOTAL: Calories 1,144 cal / **Carbs** 128 g (43%) / **Protein** 103 g (35%) / **Fat** 29 g (22%) / **Fluid** 8

1200 CALORIE MEAL PLAN

DAY 4		

Breakfast
7:00 AM

bananas	1/2 small	45 cal
whole grain rolled oats, dry	1/3 Cup(s)	100 cal
whole eggs, scrambled	2 large	182 cal
drinking water	2 Cup(s)	0 cal

MEAL TOTAL: Calories 326 cal / Carbs 32 g (40%) / Protein 13 g (16%) / Fat 16 g (44%) / Fluid 20

Snack
10:00 AM

drinking water	2 Cup(s)	0 cal
oranges	1 fruit	69 cal
peanuts, no salt, dry-roasted	2/3 oz	111 cal

MEAL TOTAL: Calories 179 cal / Carbs 22 g (44%) / Protein 6 g (12%) / Fat 10 g (44%) / Fluid 20

Lunch
12:00 PM

italian spiced pork chops	1 serving	100 cal
extra virgin olive oil	1/2 Tbsp	60 cal
balsamic vinegar	1/2 Tbsp	7 cal
tomatoes	1/4 Cup(s)	8 cal
romaine lettuce	1 Cup(s)	8 cal
whole wheat dinner rolls	1 1/2 roll	112 cal
drinking water	2 Cup(s)	0 cal

MEAL TOTAL: Calories 295 cal / Carbs 28 g (37%) / Protein 23 g (30%) / Fat 11 g (33%) / Fluid 22

Dinner
6:00 PM

wild rice, cooked	1/2 Cup(s)	83 cal
asparagus, boiled	6 spears	20 cal
beef t-bone, broiled	5 oz	268 cal
drinking water	2 Cup(s)	0 cal

MEAL TOTAL: Calories 371 cal / Carbs 21 g (23%) / Protein 42 g (46%) / Fat 13 g (31%) / Fluid 24

DAY 4 TOTAL: Calories 1,171 cal / Carbs 102 g (35%) / Protein 83 g (28%) / Fat 49 g (37%) / Fluid 86

1200 CALORIE MEAL PLAN

DAY 5

Breakfast
7:00 AM

multi-grain cheerios cereal	1 Cup(s)	120 cal
skim milk with calcium	1 1/2 Cup(s)	130 cal
drinking water	1 Cup(s)	0 cal
egg whites, cooked	2 large	34 cal

MEAL TOTAL: Calories 284 cal / **Carbs** 43 g (63%) / **Protein** 22 g (31%) / **Fat** 2 g (6%) / **Fluid** 21

Snack
10:00 AM

smooth peanut butter, no salt	1 1/2 Tbsp	141 cal
drinking water	2 Cup(s)	0 cal
apples	1/2 small	28 cal

MEAL TOTAL: Calories 169 cal / **Carbs** 12 g (26%) / **Protein** 6 g (14%) / **Fat** 12 g (60%) / **Fluid** 18

Lunch
12:00 PM

drinking water	2 Cup(s)	0 cal
whole-wheat pita bread	1 small	74 cal
turkey breast, roasted	4 oz	154 cal
tomatoes	1/4 Cup(s)	8 cal
avocados	1/4 cup	58 cal
hummus, lower sodium	3 Tbsp	78 cal

MEAL TOTAL: Calories 374 cal / **Carbs** 27 g (28%) / **Protein** 41 g (42%) / **Fat** 13 g (30%) / **Fluid** 22

Dinner
6:00 PM

mediterranean chicken	1 serving	186 cal
wild rice, cooked	2/3 Cup(s)	110 cal
cauliflower, no salt, boiled	1 Cup(s)	29 cal
drinking water	2 Cup(s)	0 cal

MEAL TOTAL: Calories 325 cal / **Carbs** 29 g (35%) / **Protein** 30 g (35%) / **Fat** 11 g (30%) / **Fluid** 26

DAY 5 TOTAL: Calories 1,151 cal / **Carbs** 112 g (38%) / **Protein** 99 g (33%) / **Fat** 38 g (29%) / **Fluid** 87

1200 CALORIE MEAL PLAN

DAY 6

Breakfast
7:00 AM

smooth peanut butter, no salt	1 1/2 Tbsp	141 cal
whole wheat mini bagel	1/2 bagel	50 cal
skim milk with calcium	1 Cup(s)	86 cal
drinking water	1 Cup(s)	0 cal
egg whites, cooked	4 large	69 cal

MEAL TOTAL: Calories 346 cal / **Carbs** 28 g (32%) / **Protein** 31 g (35%) / **Fat** 13 g (33%) / **Fluid** 20

Snack
10:00 AM

raisins, seedless	1/4 cup	123 cal
drinking water	2 Cup(s)	0 cal
cottage cheese, non-fat	1 Cup(s)	104 cal

MEAL TOTAL: Calories 228 cal / **Carbs** 42 g (71%) / **Protein** 16 g (27%) / **Fat** 1 g (2%) / **Fluid** 20

Lunch
12:00 PM

whole-wheat pita bread	1 small	74 cal
green snap beans, no salt, boiled	1/2 Cup(s)	22 cal
drinking water	2 Cup(s)	0 cal
mediterranean chicken	1 serving	186 cal

MEAL TOTAL: Calories 282 cal / **Carbs** 21 g (29%) / **Protein** 27 g (37%) / **Fat** 11 g (34%) / **Fluid** 21

Dinner
6:00 PM

drinking water	2 Cup(s)	0 cal
salmon, cooked	5 oz	217 cal
marinara spaghetti sauce, ready to serve	1/3 Cup(s)	41 cal
asparagus, boiled	4 spears	13 cal
rice penne pasta, low-carb	1 oz	104 cal

MEAL TOTAL: Calories 375 cal / **Carbs** 32 g (35%) / **Protein** 39 g (43%) / **Fat** 9 g (22%) / **Fluid** 24

DAY 6 TOTAL: Calories 1,231 cal / **Carbs** 123 g (40%) / **Protein** 114 g (36%) / **Fat** 34 g (24%) / **Fluid** 8

1200 CALORIE MEAL PLAN

DAY 7

Breakfast
7:00 AM

skim milk with calcium	1 1/2 Cup(s)	130 cal
whole wheat mini bagel	1 bagel	100 cal
whole eggs, scrambled	1 large	91 cal
drinking water	1 Cup(s)	0 cal

MEAL TOTAL: Calories 321 cal / Carbs 39 g (49%) / Protein 23 g (29%) / Fat 8 g (22%) / Fluid 21

Snack
10:00 AM

drinking water	2 Cup(s)	0 cal
celery	5 medium stalk	32 cal
smooth peanut butter, no salt	1 1/2 Tbsp	141 cal
wheat thin crackers	5 crackers	40 cal

MEAL TOTAL: Calories 213 cal / Carbs 18 g (31%) / Protein 8 g (14%) / Fat 14 g (55%) / Fluid 22

Lunch
12:00 PM

whole wheat tortillas	1 tortilla	127 cal
sliced ham, extra lean, low-sodium	4 oz	149 cal
olive oil, mayonnaise, light	1 tsp	16 cal
romaine lettuce	2 leaf	2 cal
tomatoes	1/4 Cup(s)	8 cal
iced tea, green	16 fl oz	0 cal

MEAL TOTAL: Calories 302 cal / Carbs 22 g (33%) / Protein 24 g (35%) / Fat 10 g (32%) / Fluid 21

Dinner
6:00 PM

drinking water	2 Cup(s)	0 cal
chicken, boneless, roasted	3 oz	142 cal
yams, no salt, boiled or baked	1 Cup(s)	158 cal
green snap beans, no salt, boiled	1 Cup(s)	44 cal
extra virgin olive oil	1/2 Tbsp	60 cal

MEAL TOTAL: Calories 404 cal / Carbs 47 g (46%) / Protein 26 g (25%) / Fat 13 g (29%) / Fluid 25

DAY 7 TOTAL: Calories 1,239 cal **/ Carbs** 126 g (41%) **/ Protein** 80 g (26%) **/ Fat** 44 g (33%) **/ Fluid** 89

1,600 CALORIE MEAL PLAN OUTLINES

1600 CALORIE MEAL PLAN

DAY 1

Breakfast
7:00 AM

whole eggs, poached	2 large	143 cal
oat bran, cooked	1 1/2 Cup(s)	131 cal
drinking water	1 Cup(s)	0 cal
raisins, seedless	1/4 cup	123 cal
skim milk with calcium	1 Cup(s)	86 cal

MEAL TOTAL: Calories 484 cal / **Carbs** 83 g (57%) / **Protein** 33 g (23%) / **Fat** 13 g (20%) / **Fluid** 28

Snack
10:00 AM

vanilla yogurt, low-fat	4 oz	96 cal
drinking water	2 Cup(s)	0 cal
nectarines	1 fruit	60 cal
granola oat cereal, low-fat	1/3 Cup(s)	42 cal

MEAL TOTAL: Calories 198 cal / **Carbs** 39 g (74%) / **Protein** 8 g (15%) / **Fat** 2 g (11%) / **Fluid** 23

Lunch
12:00 PM

sharp cheddar, sliced	1/2 slice	55 cal
romaine lettuce	2 leaf	2 cal
whole wheat bread	2 slice	200 cal
tomatoes	1/4 Cup(s)	8 cal
dijon mustard	1 tsp	5 cal
drinking water	2 Cup(s)	0 cal
pretzel sticks, no salt	30 pretzels	88 cal
chicken, boneless, roasted	2 oz	95 cal

MEAL TOTAL: Calories 453 cal / **Carbs** 61 g (51%) / **Protein** 31 g (26%) / **Fat** 12 g (23%) / **Fluid** 19

Dinner
6:00 PM

beef top sirloin, lean, broiled	3 oz	175 cal
extra virgin olive oil	1/2 Tbsp	60 cal
quinoa, cooked	1 Cup(s)	222 cal
drinking water	2 Cup(s)	0 cal

MEAL TOTAL: Calories 457 cal / **Carbs** 39 g (35%) / **Protein** 33 g (29%) / **Fat** 18 g (36%) / **Fluid** 22

DAY 1 TOTAL: Calories 1,592 cal / **Carbs** 222 g (52%) / **Protein** 104 g (24%) / **Fat** 45 g (24%) / **Fluid** 92

1600 CALORIE MEAL PLAN

DAY 2

Breakfast
7:00 AM

skim milk with calcium	1 Cup(s)	86 cal
drinking water	2 Cup(s)	0 cal
wheat chex cereal	1 1/2 Cup(s)	240 cal
whole eggs, poached	2 large	143 cal

MEAL TOTAL: Calories 469 cal / **Carbs** 71 g (56%) / **Protein** 31 g (24%) / **Fat** 11 g (20%) / **Fluid** 26

Snack
10:00 AM

almond butter	1 1/2 Tbsp	150 cal
drinking water	2 Cup(s)	0 cal
apples	1 small	55 cal
pretzel sticks, no salt	20 pretzels	58 cal

MEAL TOTAL: Calories 264 cal / **Carbs** 31 g (47%) / **Protein** 6 g (10%) / **Fat** 12 g (43%) / **Fluid** 19

Lunch
12:00 PM

romaine lettuce	2 leaf	2 cal
drinking water	2 Cup(s)	0 cal
baby carrots	15 large	79 cal
olive oil, mayonnaise, light	2 tsp	33 cal
tuna fish, very low-sodium, in water	4 oz	112 cal
whole-wheat pita bread	2 small	149 cal

MEAL TOTAL: Calories 374 cal / **Carbs** 50 g (52%) / **Protein** 33 g (33%) / **Fat** 7 g (15%) / **Fluid** 24

Dinner
6:00 PM

beef t-bone, broiled	3 oz	161 cal
butter, no salt	1/2 Tbsp	51 cal
drinking water	2 Cup(s)	0 cal
mustard greens, no salt, boiled	1 cup	36 cal
whole wheat dinner rolls	1 roll	74 cal
baked potato, no salt	1/2 large	139 cal

MEAL TOTAL: Calories 462 cal / **Carbs** 52 g (44%) / **Protein** 32 g (27%) / **Fat** 15 g (29%) / **Fluid** 26

DAY 2 TOTAL: Calories 1,569 cal / **Carbs** 205 g (50%) / **Protein** 102 g (25%) / **Fat** 46 g (25%) / **Fluid** 95

1600 CALORIE MEAL PLAN

DAY 3

Breakfast
7:00 AM

almond butter	2 Tbsp	200 cal
skim milk with calcium	1 Cup(s)	86 cal
drinking water	1 Cup(s)	0 cal
nectarines	1 fruit	60 cal
whole wheat bread	1 slice	100 cal

MEAL TOTAL: Calories 446 cal / **Carbs** 52 g (46%) / **Protein** 21 g (18%) / **Fat** 18 g (36%) / **Fluid** 20

Snack
10:00 AM

apples	1 small	55 cal
nut and raisin granola bars	1 bar	127 cal
drinking water	2 Cup(s)	0 cal
low-fat cottage cheese, 1%	1/2 Cup(s)	81 cal

MEAL TOTAL: Calories 264 cal / **Carbs** 36 g (53%) / **Protein** 17 g (24%) / **Fat** 7 g (23%) / **Fluid** 22

Lunch
12:00 PM

beef t-bone, broiled	3 oz	161 cal
tomatoes	1/4 Cup(s)	8 cal
romaine lettuce	2 Cup(s)	16 cal
extra virgin olive oil	1/2 Tbsp	60 cal
balsamic vinegar	1/2 Tbsp	7 cal
whole wheat dinner rolls	1 roll	74 cal
iced tea, green	16 fl oz	0 cal
quinoa, cooked	1/2 Cup(s)	111 cal

MEAL TOTAL: Calories 437 cal / **Carbs** 40 g (37%) / **Protein** 30 g (27%) / **Fat** 18 g (36%) / **Fluid** 25

Dinner
6:00 PM

whole-wheat pita bread	1 small	74 cal
drinking water	2 Cup(s)	0 cal
summer squash, no salt, boiled	2 cup	72 cal
wild rice, cooked	3/4 Cup(s)	124 cal
chicken & quinoa with vegetables	1 serving	217 cal

MEAL TOTAL: Calories 488 cal / **Carbs** 80 g (63%) / **Protein** 33 g (26%) / **Fat** 6 g (11%) / **Fluid** 36

DAY 3 TOTAL: Calories 1,635 cal / **Carbs** 208 g (50%) / **Protein** 100 g (24%) / **Fat** 49 g (26%) / **Fluid** 102

1600 CALORIE MEAL PLAN

DAY 4

Breakfast
7:00 AM

salsa, ready to serve	2 Tbsp	10 cal
whole eggs, scrambled	2 large	182 cal
whole wheat tortillas	1 tortilla	127 cal
drinking water	1 Cup(s)	0 cal
orange juice	1 Cup(s)	112 cal

MEAL TOTAL: Calories 430 cal / Carbs 49 g (45%) / Protein 18 g (17%) / Fat 18 g (38%) / Fluid 20

Snack
10:00 AM

low-fat cottage cheese, 1%	3/4 Cup(s)	122 cal
drinking water	2 Cup(s)	0 cal
nectarines	1 fruit	60 cal
pretzel sticks, no salt	15 pretzels	44 cal

MEAL TOTAL: Calories 226 cal / Carbs 28 g (50%) / Protein 24 g (41%) / Fat 2 g (9%) / Fluid 25

Lunch
12:00 PM

butter, no salt	1/2 Tbsp	51 cal
quinoa, cooked	1/2 Cup(s)	111 cal
drinking water	2 Cup(s)	0 cal
mixed vegetables, frozen no salt, boiled	1 Cup(s)	59 cal
chicken & quinoa with vegetables	1 serving	217 cal

MEAL TOTAL: Calories 438 cal / Carbs 54 g (50%) / Protein 29 g (26%) / Fat 12 g (24%) / Fluid 26

Dinner
6:00 PM

pork tenderloin, lean, cooked	3 oz	122 cal
drinking water	2 Cup(s)	0 cal
mustard greens, no salt, boiled	1/2 cup	18 cal
navy beans, no salt, boiled	1/2 Cup(s)	127 cal
wild rice, cooked	1 Cup(s)	166 cal

MEAL TOTAL: Calories 433 cal / Carbs 62 g (56%) / Protein 38 g (35%) / Fat 4 g (9%) / Fluid 26

DAY 4 TOTAL: Calories 1,527 cal / Carbs 193 g (51%) / Protein 109 g (28%) / Fat 36 g (21%) / Fluid 97

1600 CALORIE MEAL PLAN

DAY 5

Breakfast
7:00 AM

wheat chex cereal	1 Cup(s)	160 cal
skim milk with calcium	1 Cup(s)	86 cal
drinking water	2 Cup(s)	0 cal
bacon, low-sodium, cooked	2 slice cooked	87 cal
whole eggs, scrambled	1 large	91 cal

MEAL TOTAL: Calories 424 cal / **Carbs** 52 g (46%) / **Protein** 27 g (24%) / **Fat** 15 g (30%) / Fluid 25

Snack
10:00 AM

apples	1 small	55 cal
drinking water	2 Cup(s)	0 cal
almond butter	1 1/2 Tbsp	150 cal

MEAL TOTAL: Calories 205 cal / **Carbs** 19 g (37%) / **Protein** 5 g (9%) / **Fat** 12 g (54%) / Fluid 19

Lunch
12:00 PM

extra virgin olive oil	1/2 Tbsp	60 cal
balsamic vinegar	1/2 Tbsp	7 cal
romaine lettuce	2 Cup(s)	16 cal
drinking water	2 Cup(s)	0 cal
pork tenderloin, lean, cooked	5 oz	203 cal
whole wheat dinner rolls	1 roll	74 cal
baked potato, no salt	1/2 large	139 cal

MEAL TOTAL: Calories 499 cal / **Carbs** 50 g (40%) / **Protein** 44 g (35%) / **Fat** 14 g (25%) / Fluid 27

Dinner
6:00 PM

chopped kale salad with chicken	1 serving	262 cal
whole-wheat pita bread	1 1/2 small	112 cal
drinking water	2 Cup(s)	0 cal

MEAL TOTAL: Calories 374 cal / **Carbs** 33 g (34%) / **Protein** 37 g (38%) / **Fat** 12 g (28%) / Fluid 22

DAY 5 TOTAL: Calories 1,502 cal **/ Carbs** 155 g (40%) **/ Protein** 113 g (29%) **/ Fat** 53 g (31%) **/ Fluid** 93

1600 CALORIE MEAL PLAN

DAY 6

Breakfast
7:00 AM

drinking water	1 Cup(s)	0 cal
bananas	1 small	90 cal
almond butter	1 Tbsp	100 cal
whole wheat bread	2 slice	200 cal
skim milk with calcium	1 Cup(s)	86 cal

MEAL TOTAL: Calories 476 cal / **Carbs** 78 g (61%) / **Protein** 22 g (18%) / **Fat** 12 g (21%) / **Fluid** 18

Snack
10:00 AM

nectarines	1 fruit	60 cal
drinking water	2 Cup(s)	0 cal
vanilla yogurt, low-fat	6 oz	145 cal

MEAL TOTAL: Calories 204 cal / **Carbs** 38 g (71%) / **Protein** 10 g (18%) / **Fat** 3 g (11%) / **Fluid** 25

Lunch
12:00 PM

butter, no salt	1/2 Tbsp	51 cal
whole wheat dinner rolls	1 1/2 roll	112 cal
iced tea, green	16 fl oz	0 cal
chopped kale salad with chicken	1 serving	262 cal

MEAL TOTAL: Calories 425 cal / **Carbs** 31 g (29%) / **Protein** 36 g (33%) / **Fat** 19 g (38%) / **Fluid** 22

Dinner
6:00 PM

butter, no salt	1/2 Tbsp	51 cal
wild rice, cooked	1 1/3 Cup(s)	221 cal
drinking water	2 Cup(s)	0 cal
summer squash, no salt, boiled	1 cup	36 cal
salmon, cooked	4 oz	174 cal

MEAL TOTAL: Calories 482 cal / **Carbs** 54 g (45%) / **Protein** 38 g (31%) / **Fat** 13 g (24%) / **Fluid** 30

DAY 6 TOTAL: Calories 1,587 cal / **Carbs** 202 g (49%) / **Protein** 107 g (26%) / **Fat** 46 g (25%) / **Fluid** 95

1600 CALORIE MEAL PLAN

DAY 7

Breakfast
7:00 AM

drinking water	1 Cup(s)	0 cal
whole eggs, poached	1 large	72 cal
whole wheat bread	2 slice	200 cal
skim milk with calcium	1 Cup(s)	86 cal
nectarines	1 fruit	60 cal

MEAL TOTAL: Calories 418 cal / Carbs 67 g (60%) / Protein 26 g (23%) / Fat 9 g (17%) / Fluid 21

Snack
10:00 AM

drinking water	2 Cup(s)	0 cal
baby carrots	15 large	79 cal
hummus, lower sodium	2 Tbsp	52 cal
pretzel sticks, no salt	30 pretzels	88 cal

MEAL TOTAL: Calories 219 cal / Carbs 42 g (74%) / Protein 6 g (11%) / Fat 4 g (15%) / Fluid 24

Lunch
12:00 PM

romaine lettuce	2 leaf	2 cal
whole wheat tortillas	2 tortilla	254 cal
dijon mustard	2 tsp	10 cal
tomatoes	1/4 Cup(s)	8 cal
drinking water	2 Cup(s)	0 cal
turkey breast, roasted	4 oz	154 cal
olive oil, mayonnaise, light	2 tsp	33 cal

MEAL TOTAL: Calories 461 cal / Carbs 40 g (36%) / Protein 42 g (37%) / Fat 14 g (27%) / Fluid 21

Dinner
6:00 PM

chicken, boneless, roasted	3 oz	142 cal
quinoa, cooked	1 Cup(s)	222 cal
drinking water	2 Cup(s)	0 cal
brussels sprouts, no salt, boiled	1 Cup(s)	28 cal
butter, no salt	1/2 Tbsp	51 cal

MEAL TOTAL: Calories 443 cal / Carbs 45 g (41%) / Protein 31 g (28%) / Fat 15 g (31%) / Fluid 25

DAY 7 TOTAL: Calories 1,541 cal / **Carbs** 194 g (49%) / **Protein** 106 g (27%) / **Fat** 41 g (24%) / **Fluid** 91

2,000 CALORIE MEAL PLAN OUTLINES

2000 CALORIE MEAL PLAN

DAY 1

Breakfast
7:00 AM

whole eggs, scrambled	1 large	91 cal
blueberries	1/2 Cup(s)	41 cal
oatmeal, steel cut	2/3 Cup(s)	400 cal
drinking water	2 Cup(s)	0 cal

MEAL TOTAL: Calories 532 cal / **Carbs** 83 g (62%) / **Protein** 20 g (15%) / **Fat** 14 g (23%) / **Fluid** 20

Snack
10:00 AM

tangerines/ mandarin oranges	1 medium	45 cal
low-fat cottage cheese, 1%	1 Cup(s)	163 cal
coconut water	1 Cup(s)	46 cal
drinking water	1 Cup(s)	0 cal

MEAL TOTAL: Calories 253 cal / **Carbs** 26 g (41%) / **Protein** 30 g (48%) / **Fat** 3 g (11%) / **Fluid** 24

Lunch
12:00 PM

triscuit crackers, light salt	10 crackers	200 cal
baby carrots	5 large	26 cal
tomatoes	1/4 Cup(s)	8 cal
iced tea, green	16 fl oz	0 cal
whole wheat dinner rolls	2 roll	149 cal
turkey breast, roasted	2 oz	77 cal
dijon mustard	1 tsp	5 cal

MEAL TOTAL: Calories 465 cal / **Carbs** 70 g (57%) / **Protein** 27 g (23%) / **Fat** 11 g (20%) / **Fluid** 22

Snack
3:00 PM

skim milk with calcium	1 Cup(s)	86 cal
honey peanut yogurt balance bar	1 bar	200 cal
drinking water	1 Cup(s)	0 cal

MEAL TOTAL: Calories 286 cal / **Carbs** 34 g (45%) / **Protein** 23 g (32%) / **Fat** 7 g (23%) / **Fluid** 16

Dinner
6:00 PM

orange roughy fish, cooked	3 oz	89 cal
drinking water	2 Cup(s)	0 cal
mixed vegetables, frozen no salt, boiled	1 Cup(s)	59 cal
wild rice, cooked	1 Cup(s)	166 cal
extra virgin olive oil	1 Tbsp	120 cal

MEAL TOTAL: Calories 434 cal / **Carbs** 47 g (42%) / **Protein** 28 g (26%) / **Fat** 15 g (32%) / **Fluid** 25

DAY 1 TOTAL: Calories 1,971 cal / **Carbs** 261 g (52%) / **Protein** 130 g (26%) / **Fat** 50 g (22%) / **Fluid** 106

2000 CALORIE MEAL PLAN

DAY 2			

Breakfast
7:00 AM

skim milk with calcium	2 Cup(s)	173 cal
kashi golean crunch cereal	1 3/4 Cup(s)	339 cal
drinking water	1 Cup(s)	0 cal
whole eggs, scrambled	1 large	91 cal

MEAL TOTAL: Calories 602 cal / Carbs 93 g (58%) / Protein 38 g (24%) / Fat 13 g (18%) / Fluid 25

Snack
10:00 AM

apples	1 large	110 cal
honey peanut yogurt balance bar	1 bar	200 cal
drinking water	2 Cup(s)	0 cal

MEAL TOTAL: Calories 310 cal / Carbs 51 g (61%) / Protein 16 g (19%) / Fat 7 g (20%) / Fluid 22

Lunch
12:00 PM

drinking water	2 Cup(s)	0 cal
avocados	1/3 cup	78 cal
salsa, ready to serve	1 Tbsp	5 cal
whole wheat tortillas	2 tortilla	254 cal
black beans, no salt, boiled	1/2 Cup(s)	114 cal

MEAL TOTAL: Calories 450 cal / Carbs 63 g (54%) / Protein 17 g (15%) / Fat 16 g (31%) / Fluid 20

Snack
3:00 PM

fruit yogurt, non-fat	1/2 cup	116 cal
drinking water	2 Cup(s)	0 cal
bananas	1 small	90 cal

MEAL TOTAL: Calories 206 cal / Carbs 46 g (86%) / Protein 6 g (12%) / Fat 1 g (2%) / Fluid 22

Dinner
6:00 PM

chicken, boneless, roasted	6 oz	284 cal
peas & carrots, no salt, boiled	1/2 Cup(s)	19 cal
barley, cooked	1 Cup(s)	193 cal
drinking water	2 Cup(s)	0 cal
romaine lettuce	1 Cup(s)	8 cal
balsamic vinaigrette salad dressing	1 Tbsp	35 cal

MEAL TOTAL: Calories 539 cal / Carbs 52 g (38%) / Protein 48 g (36%) / Fat 15 g (26%) / Fluid 26

DAY 2 TOTAL: Calories 2,109 cal / **Carbs** 305 g (56%) / **Protein** 125 g (23%) / **Fat** 52 g (21%) / **Fluid** 115

2000 CALORIE MEAL PLAN

DAY 3

Breakfast
7:00 AM

drinking water	1 Cup(s)	0 cal
orange juice	1 Cup(s)	112 cal
whole wheat english muffin	2 muffin	268 cal
smooth peanut butter, no salt	1 1/2 Tbsp	141 cal

MEAL TOTAL: Calories 521 cal / **Carbs** 84 g (61%) / **Protein** 19 g (14%) / Fat 15 g (25%) / Fluid 17

Snack
10:00 AM

honey peanut yogurt balance bar	1 bar	200 cal
bananas	1 small	90 cal
drinking water	2 Cup(s)	0 cal

MEAL TOTAL: Calories 290 cal / **Carbs** 45 g (58%) / **Protein** 16 g (21%) / Fat 7 g (21%) / Fluid 19

Lunch
12:00 PM

dijon mustard	1 tsp	5 cal
romaine lettuce	2 leaf	2 cal
whole wheat tortillas	1 tortilla	127 cal
chicken, boneless, roasted	5 oz	237 cal
iced tea, green	16 fl oz	0 cal
olive oil, mayonnaise, light	1/2 Tbsp	25 cal
apples	1 large	110 cal

MEAL TOTAL: Calories 506 cal / **Carbs** 49 g (39%) / **Protein** 40 g (32%) / Fat 16 g (29%) / Fluid 26

Snack
3:00 PM

triscuit crackers, light salt	5 crackers	100 cal
drinking water	2 Cup(s)	0 cal
baby carrots	10 large	53 cal
hummus, lower sodium	3 Tbsp	78 cal

MEAL TOTAL: Calories 231 cal / **Carbs** 36 g (58%) / **Protein** 7 g (12%) / Fat 8 g (30%) / Fluid 22

Dinner
6:00 PM

skim milk with calcium	1 1/2 Cup(s)	130 cal
drinking water	1 Cup(s)	0 cal
beef & broccoli with brown rice	1 serving	310 cal

MEAL TOTAL: Calories 439 cal / **Carbs** 50 g (46%) / **Protein** 34 g (32%) / Fat 11 g (22%) / Fluid 26

DAY 3 TOTAL: Calories 1,986 cal / **Carbs** 264 g (52%) / **Protein** 117 g (23%) / **Fat** 58 g (25%) / **Fluid** 109

2000 CALORIE MEAL PLAN

DAY 4

Breakfast
7:00 AM

almonds, slivered	1/3 oz	51 cal
blueberries	1/2 Cup(s)	41 cal
oatmeal, steel cut	2/3 Cup(s)	400 cal
drinking water	1 Cup(s)	0 cal
skim milk with calcium	1 Cup(s)	86 cal

MEAL TOTAL: Calories 579 cal / **Carbs** 98 g (67%) / **Protein** 24 g (17%) / **Fat** 10 g (16%) / **Fluid** 18

Snack
10:00 AM

low-fat cottage cheese, 1%	1/2 Cup(s)	81 cal
blackberries	1 Cup(s)	62 cal
coconut water	2 Cup(s)	91 cal

MEAL TOTAL: Calories 234 cal / **Carbs** 35 g (58%) / **Protein** 19 g (32%) / **Fat** 3 g (10%) / **Fluid** 23

Lunch
12:00 PM

beef & broccoli with brown rice	1 serving	310 cal
balsamic vinaigrette salad dressing	1 Tbsp	35 cal
romaine lettuce	1 Cup(s)	8 cal
drinking water	2 Cup(s)	0 cal
extra virgin olive oil	3/4 Tbsp	90 cal

MEAL TOTAL: Calories 443 cal / **Carbs** 36 g (32%) / **Protein** 22 g (20%) / **Fat** 24 g (48%) / **Fluid** 24

Snack
3:00 PM

honey peanut yogurt balance bar	1 bar	200 cal
cucumber	1 cucumber	45 cal
drinking water	2 Cup(s)	0 cal

MEAL TOTAL: Calories 245 cal / **Carbs** 33 g (49%) / **Protein** 17 g (26%) / **Fat** 7 g (25%) / **Fluid** 26

Dinner
6:00 PM

mixed vegetables, frozen no salt, boiled	1 1/3 Cup(s)	79 cal
pork tenderloin, lean, cooked	5 oz	203 cal
drinking water	2 Cup(s)	0 cal
whole wheat dinner rolls	3 roll	223 cal

MEAL TOTAL: Calories 505 cal / **Carbs** 59 g (46%) / **Protein** 48 g (38%) / **Fat** 9 g (16%) / **Fluid** 24

DAY 4 TOTAL: Calories 2,006 cal / **Carbs** 260 g (51%) / **Protein** 131 g (26%) / **Fat** 53 g (23%) / **Fluid** 114

2000 CALORIE MEAL PLAN

DAY 5

Breakfast
7:00 AM

kashi golean crunch cereal	1 1/2 Cup(s)	290 cal
skim milk with calcium	1 1/2 Cup(s)	130 cal
apricots	3 apricot	50 cal

MEAL TOTAL: Calories 470 cal / Carbs 88 g (69%) / Protein 27 g (21%) / Fat 6 g (10%) / Fluid 15

Snack
10:00 AM

blueberries	1 Cup(s)	83 cal
almonds, slivered	1/2 oz	77 cal
low-fat cottage cheese, 1%	1 Cup(s)	163 cal
drinking water	2 Cup(s)	0 cal

MEAL TOTAL: Calories 322 cal / Carbs 33 g (40%) / Protein 32 g (40%) / Fat 7 g (20%) / Fluid 26

Lunch
12:00 PM

dijon mustard	1 tsp	5 cal
whole wheat dinner rolls	3 roll	223 cal
sliced ham, extra lean, low-sodium	4 slices	110 cal
balsamic vinaigrette salad dressing	1 1/2 Tbsp	53 cal
tomatoes	1/4 Cup(s)	8 cal
romaine lettuce	1 Cup(s)	8 cal
drinking water	2 Cup(s)	0 cal
pretzel sticks, no salt	1/2 oz	54 cal

MEAL TOTAL: Calories 461 cal / Carbs 61 g (55%) / Protein 24 g (21%) / Fat 12 g (24%) / Fluid 22

Snack
3:00 PM

triscuit crackers, light salt	8 crackers	160 cal
hummus, lower sodium	3 Tbsp	78 cal
drinking water	2 Cup(s)	0 cal

MEAL TOTAL: Calories 238 cal / Carbs 33 g (53%) / Protein 8 g (12%) / Fat 10 g (35%) / Fluid 17

Dinner
6:00 PM

chicken, boneless, roasted	5 oz	237 cal
drinking water	2 Cup(s)	0 cal
adzuki bean salad	1 serving	219 cal

MEAL TOTAL: Calories 456 cal / Carbs 31 g (27%) / Protein 45 g (40%) / Fat 17 g (33%) / Fluid 22

DAY 5 TOTAL: Calories 1,947 cal / Carbs 246 g (50%) / Protein 136 g (27%) / Fat 51 g (23%) / Fluid 102

2000 CALORIE MEAL PLAN

DAY 6

Breakfast
7:00 AM

drinking water	2 Cup(s)	0 cal
whole wheat tortillas	3 tortilla	381 cal
salsa, ready to serve	2 Tbsp	10 cal
whole eggs, scrambled	1 large	91 cal
avocados	1/3 cup	78 cal

MEAL TOTAL: Calories 560 cal / **Carbs** 64 g (45%) / **Protein** 20 g (14%) / **Fat** 26 g (41%) / **Fluid** 21

Snack
10:00 AM

bananas	1 1/2 small	135 cal
low-fat cottage cheese, 1%	1/2 Cup(s)	81 cal
drinking water	2 Cup(s)	0 cal

MEAL TOTAL: Calories 216 cal / **Carbs** 38 g (66%) / **Protein** 16 g (27%) / **Fat** 2 g (7%) / **Fluid** 23

Lunch
12:00 PM

turkey breast, roasted	3 oz	116 cal
drinking water	2 Cup(s)	0 cal
adzuki bean salad	1 serving	219 cal

MEAL TOTAL: Calories 335 cal / **Carbs** 31 g (36%) / **Protein** 34 g (40%) / **Fat** 9 g (24%) / **Fluid** 21

Snack
3:00 PM

skim milk with calcium	1 1/2 Cup(s)	130 cal
smooth peanut butter, no salt	1/2 Tbsp	47 cal
apples	1 large	110 cal
drinking water	1 Cup(s)	0 cal

MEAL TOTAL: Calories 287 cal / **Carbs** 49 g (65%) / **Protein** 15 g (20%) / **Fat** 5 g (15%) / **Fluid** 26

Dinner
6:00 PM

spinach, no salt, boiled	2 Cup(s)	83 cal
drinking water	2 Cup(s)	0 cal
salmon, cooked	2 oz	87 cal
parmesan cheese, shredded	1/2 Tbsp	10 cal
macaroni, cooked	2 Cup(s)	347 cal

MEAL TOTAL: Calories 527 cal / **Carbs** 88 g (62%) / **Protein** 40 g (28%) / **Fat** 6 g (10%) / **Fluid** 35

DAY 6 TOTAL: Calories 1,925 cal / **Carbs** 269 g (54%) / **Protein** 125 g (25%) / **Fat** 48 g (21%) / **Fluid** 125

2000 CALORIE MEAL PLAN

DAY 7

Breakfast
7:00 AM

orange juice	1/2 Cup(s)	56 cal
whole eggs, scrambled	1 large	91 cal
whole wheat english muffin	1 1/2 muffin	201 cal
skim milk with calcium	2 Cup(s)	173 cal

MEAL TOTAL: Calories 521 cal / **Carbs** 78 g (59%) / **Protein** 32 g (24%) / **Fat** 10 g (17%) / **Fluid** 22

Snack
10:00 AM

drinking water	2 Cup(s)	0 cal
fruit yogurt, non-fat	3/4 cup	175 cal
coconut water	1 Cup(s)	46 cal
bananas	1 small	90 cal

MEAL TOTAL: Calories 310 cal / **Carbs** 67 g (83%) / **Protein** 11 g (14%) / **Fat** 1 g (3%) / **Fluid** 31

Lunch
12:00 PM

iced tea, green	16 fl oz	0 cal
dijon mustard	1 tsp	5 cal
romaine lettuce	3 leaf	3 cal
turkey breast, roasted	2 oz	77 cal
whole wheat tortillas	3 tortilla	381 cal
pretzel sticks, no salt	1 oz	108 cal

MEAL TOTAL: Calories 574 cal / **Carbs** 80 g (56%) / **Protein** 32 g (22%) / **Fat** 14 g (22%) / **Fluid** 19

Snack
3:00 PM

baby carrots	10 large	53 cal
drinking water	2 Cup(s)	0 cal
hummus, lower sodium	2 Tbsp	52 cal
triscuit crackers, light salt	8 crackers	160 cal

MEAL TOTAL: Calories 265 cal / **Carbs** 44 g (62%) / **Protein** 7 g (11%) / **Fat** 9 g (27%) / **Fluid** 21

Dinner
6:00 PM

barley, cooked	2/3 Cup(s)	129 cal
balsamic vinaigrette salad dressing	1 Tbsp	35 cal
drinking water	2 Cup(s)	0 cal
chicken, boneless, roasted	2 oz	95 cal
peas & carrots, no salt, boiled	1 Cup(s)	38 cal
romaine lettuce	1 Cup(s)	8 cal
extra virgin olive oil	3/4 Tbsp	90 cal

MEAL TOTAL: Calories 395 cal / **Carbs** 41 g (41%) / **Protein** 20 g (19%) / **Fat** 18 g (40%) / **Fluid** 24

DAY 7 TOTAL: Calories 2,064 cal / **Carbs** 309 g (59%) / **Protein** 102 g (19%) / **Fat** 52 g (22%) / **Fluid** 117

2,400 CALORIE MEAL PLAN OUTLINES

2400 CALORIE MEAL PLAN

DAY 1

Breakfast
7:00 AM

raisins, seedless	1/4 cup	123 cal
whole eggs, poached	1 large	72 cal
drinking water	1 Cup(s)	0 cal
orange juice	1 Cup(s)	112 cal
oat bran, cooked	2 Cup(s)	175 cal

MEAL TOTAL: Calories 482 cal **/ Carbs** 109 g (71%) **/ Protein** 23 g (15%) **/ Fat** 9 g (14%) **/ Fluid** 29

Snack
10:00 AM

nectarines	1 fruit	60 cal
vanilla yogurt, low-fat	8 oz	193 cal
drinking water	1 Cup(s)	0 cal
granola oat cereal, low-fat	2/3 Cup(s)	84 cal

MEAL TOTAL: Calories 337 cal **/ Carbs** 64 g (73%) **/ Protein** 14 g (16%) **/ Fat** 4 g (11%) **/ Fluid** 18

Lunch
12:00 PM

chicken, boneless, roasted	3 oz	142 cal
pretzel sticks, no salt	30 pretzels	88 cal
sharp cheddar, sliced	2 slice	220 cal
romaine lettuce	2 leaf	2 cal
whole wheat bread	2 slice	200 cal
tomatoes	1/2 Cup(s)	16 cal
dijon mustard	2 tsp	10 cal
drinking water	2 Cup(s)	0 cal
olive oil, mayonnaise, light	2 tsp	33 cal

MEAL TOTAL: Calories 711 cal **/ Carbs** 63 g (35%) **/ Protein** 49 g (27%) **/ Fat** 31 g (38%) **/ Fluid** 21

Snack
3:00 PM

nut and raisin granola bars	1 bar	127 cal
drinking water	1 Cup(s)	0 cal
bananas	1 small	90 cal
skim milk with calcium	1 Cup(s)	86 cal

MEAL TOTAL: Calories 303 cal **/ Carbs** 53 g (67%) **/ Protein** 12 g (15%) **/ Fat** 6 g (18%) **/ Fluid** 18

Dinner
6:00 PM

halibut fish, cooked	4 oz	126 cal
drinking water	2 Cup(s)	0 cal
quinoa, cooked	1 1/2 Cup(s)	333 cal
extra virgin olive oil	1/2 Tbsp	60 cal
brussels sprouts, no salt, boiled	1 Cup(s)	28 cal

MEAL TOTAL: Calories 547 cal **/ Carbs** 65 g (47%) **/ Protein** 40 g (29%) **/ Fat** 15 g (24%) **/ Fluid** 28

DAY 1 TOTAL: Calories 2,379 cal **/ Carbs** 353 g (55%) **/ Protein** 138 g (22%) **/ Fat** 65 g (23%) **/ Fluid** 115

2400 CALORIE MEAL PLAN

DAY 2

Breakfast
7:00 AM

skim milk with calcium	2 Cup(s)	173 cal
whole eggs, poached	3 large	215 cal
drinking water	2 Cup(s)	0 cal
wheat chex cereal	2 Cup(s)	320 cal

MEAL TOTAL: **Calories** 707 cal / **Carbs** 103 g (54%) / **Protein** 49 g (26%) / **Fat** 17 g (20%) / **Fluid** 35

Snack
10:00 AM

almond butter	1 1/2 Tbsp	150 cal
drinking water	2 Cup(s)	0 cal
apples	1 small	55 cal
pretzel sticks, no salt	35 pretzels	102 cal

MEAL TOTAL: **Calories** 307 cal / **Carbs** 41 g (53%) / **Protein** 7 g (10%) / **Fat** 13 g (37%) / **Fluid** 19

Lunch
12:00 PM

romaine lettuce	2 leaf	2 cal
drinking water	2 Cup(s)	0 cal
baby carrots	15 large	79 cal
olive oil, mayonnaise, light	2 tsp	33 cal
whole-wheat pita bread	2 small	149 cal
tuna fish, very low-sodium, in water	4 oz	112 cal
triscuit crackers, light salt	10 crackers	200 cal

MEAL TOTAL: **Calories** 574 cal / **Carbs** 84 g (55%) / **Protein** 38 g (25%) / **Fat** 13 g (20%) / **Fluid** 24

Snack
3:00 PM

nut and raisin granola bars	1 bar	127 cal
drinking water	2 Cup(s)	0 cal
nectarines	1 fruit	60 cal
low-fat cottage cheese, 1%	1 Cup(s)	163 cal

MEAL TOTAL: **Calories** 350 cal / **Carbs** 38 g (43%) / **Protein** 32 g (36%) / **Fat** 8 g (21%) / **Fluid** 26

Dinner
6:00 PM

beef t-bone, broiled	3 oz	161 cal
drinking water	2 Cup(s)	0 cal
butter, no salt	1/2 Tbsp	51 cal
mustard greens, no salt, boiled	2/3 cup	24 cal
baked potato, no salt	1/2 large	139 cal
whole wheat dinner rolls	1 roll	74 cal

MEAL TOTAL: **Calories** 450 cal / **Carbs** 50 g (43%) / **Protein** 31 g (27%) / **Fat** 15 g (30%) / **Fluid** 25

DAY 2 TOTAL: Calories 2,389 cal / **Carbs** 316 g (51%) / **Protein** 157 g (25%) / **Fat** 67 g (24%) / **Fluid** 129

2400 CALORIE MEAL PLAN

DAY 3

Breakfast
7:00 AM

almond butter	2 Tbsp	200 cal
skim milk with calcium	1 Cup(s)	86 cal
nectarines	1 fruit	60 cal
drinking water	1 Cup(s)	0 cal
whole wheat bread	2 slice	200 cal

MEAL TOTAL: Calories 546 cal / **Carbs** 72 g (51%) / **Protein** 26 g (18%) / **Fat** 20 g (31%) / Fluid 20

Snack
10:00 AM

drinking water	2 Cup(s)	0 cal
nut and raisin granola bars	1 bar	127 cal
apples	1 small	55 cal
low-fat cottage cheese, 1%	3/4 Cup(s)	122 cal

MEAL TOTAL: Calories 304 cal / **Carbs** 37 g (48%) / **Protein** 24 g (30%) / **Fat** 8 g (22%) / Fluid 24

Lunch
12:00 PM

balsamic vinegar	1/2 Tbsp	7 cal
extra virgin olive oil	1/2 Tbsp	60 cal
romaine lettuce	2 Cup(s)	16 cal
tomatoes	1/4 Cup(s)	8 cal
beef t-bone, broiled	3 oz	161 cal
iced tea, green	16 fl oz	0 cal
quinoa, cooked	1 Cup(s)	222 cal
whole wheat dinner rolls	1 roll	74 cal

MEAL TOTAL: Calories 548 cal / **Carbs** 60 g (43%) / **Protein** 34 g (25%) / **Fat** 20 g (32%) / Fluid 27

Snack
3:00 PM

pretzel sticks, no salt	30 pretzels	88 cal
baby carrots	15 large	79 cal
drinking water	2 Cup(s)	0 cal
hummus, lower sodium	3 Tbsp	78 cal

MEAL TOTAL: Calories 245 cal / **Carbs** 44 g (69%) / **Protein** 7 g (12%) / **Fat** 5 g (19%) / Fluid 24

Dinner
6:00 PM

wild rice, cooked	2 Cup(s)	331 cal
whole-wheat pita bread	1 small	74 cal
drinking water	2 Cup(s)	0 cal
summer squash, no salt, boiled	1 cup	36 cal
chicken & quinoa with vegetables	1 1/2 serving	325 cal

MEAL TOTAL: Calories 767 cal / **Carbs** 127 g (65%) / **Protein** 50 g (26%) / **Fat** 8 g (9%) / Fluid 37

DAY 3 TOTAL: Calories 2,411 cal / **Carbs** 340 g (55%) / **Protein** 141 g (23%) / **Fat** 61 g (22%) / **Fluid** 132

2400 CALORIE MEAL PLAN

DAY 4

Breakfast
7:00 AM

orange juice	1 Cup(s)	112 cal
drinking water	1 Cup(s)	0 cal
whole wheat tortillas	3 tortilla	381 cal
salsa, ready to serve	2 Tbsp	10 cal
whole eggs, scrambled	1 large	91 cal

MEAL TOTAL: Calories 593 cal / Carbs 85 g (57%) / Protein 20 g (14%) / Fat 19 g (29%) / Fluid 19

Snack
10:00 AM

low-fat cottage cheese, 1%	1 Cup(s)	163 cal
pretzel sticks, no salt	20 pretzels	58 cal
drinking water	2 Cup(s)	0 cal
nectarines	1 fruit	60 cal

MEAL TOTAL: Calories 281 cal / Carbs 33 g (46%) / Protein 31 g (44%) / Fat 3 g (10%) / Fluid 26

Lunch
12:00 PM

whole wheat dinner rolls	1 roll	74 cal
drinking water	2 Cup(s)	0 cal
mixed vegetables, frozen no salt, boiled	3/4 Cup(s)	44 cal
quinoa, cooked	1/3 Cup(s)	74 cal
butter, no salt	1/2 Tbsp	51 cal
chicken & quinoa with vegetables	1 1/2 serving	325 cal

MEAL TOTAL: Calories 569 cal / Carbs 70 g (50%) / Protein 40 g (28%) / Fat 14 g (22%) / Fluid 27

Snack
3:00 PM

drinking water	1 Cup(s)	0 cal
nut and raisin granola bars	1 bar	127 cal
skim milk with calcium	1 Cup(s)	86 cal
raisins, seedless	1/4 cup	123 cal

MEAL TOTAL: Calories 337 cal / Carbs 62 g (71%) / Protein 12 g (13%) / Fat 6 g (16%) / Fluid 16

Dinner
6:00 PM

navy beans, no salt, boiled	3/4 Cup(s)	191 cal
pork tenderloin, lean, cooked	4 oz	162 cal
mustard greens, no salt, boiled	3/4 cup	27 cal
drinking water	2 Cup(s)	0 cal
wild rice, cooked	1 1/4 Cup(s)	207 cal

MEAL TOTAL: Calories 588 cal / Carbs 84 g (56%) / Protein 52 g (35%) / Fat 6 g (9%) / Fluid 30

DAY 4 TOTAL: Calories 2,368 cal / **Carbs** 335 g (56%) / **Protein** 155 g (26%) / **Fat** 49 g (18%) / **Fluid** 118

2400 CALORIE MEAL PLAN

DAY 5

Breakfast
7:00 AM

drinking water	2 Cup(s)	0 cal
bacon, low-sodium, cooked	2 slice cooked	87 cal
whole eggs, scrambled	1 large	91 cal
skim milk with calcium	2 Cup(s)	173 cal
wheat chex cereal	1 1/2 Cup(s)	240 cal

MEAL TOTAL: Calories 590 cal / **Carbs** 84 g (53%) / **Protein** 39 g (25%) / **Fat** 16 g (22%) / **Fluid** 33

Snack
10:00 AM

drinking water	2 Cup(s)	0 cal
almond butter	2 Tbsp	200 cal
apples	1 small	55 cal
triscuit crackers, light salt	10 crackers	200 cal

MEAL TOTAL: Calories 455 cal / **Carbs** 54 g (46%) / **Protein** 11 g (10%) / **Fat** 23 g (44%) / **Fluid** 19

Lunch
12:00 PM

romaine lettuce	2 Cup(s)	16 cal
extra virgin olive oil	1/2 Tbsp	60 cal
drinking water	2 Cup(s)	0 cal
pork tenderloin, lean, cooked	4 oz	162 cal
whole wheat dinner rolls	1 roll	74 cal
baked potato, no salt	3/4 large	209 cal
balsamic vinegar	1/2 Tbsp	7 cal

MEAL TOTAL: Calories 528 cal / **Carbs** 66 g (49%) / **Protein** 39 g (29%) / **Fat** 13 g (22%) / **Fluid** 28

Snack
3:00 PM

baby carrots	20 large	105 cal
drinking water	2 Cup(s)	0 cal
hummus, lower sodium	2 Tbsp	52 cal
pretzel sticks, no salt	40 pretzels	117 cal

MEAL TOTAL: Calories 274 cal / **Carbs** 54 g (76%) / **Protein** 7 g (11%) / **Fat** 4 g (13%) / **Fluid** 26

Dinner
6:00 PM

chopped kale salad with chicken	1 serving	262 cal
whole-wheat pita bread	2 small	149 cal
drinking water	2 Cup(s)	0 cal

MEAL TOTAL: Calories 411 cal / **Carbs** 41 g (38%) / **Protein** 38 g (36%) / **Fat** 12 g (26%) / **Fluid** 22

DAY 5 TOTAL: Calories 2,259 cal / **Carbs** 298 g (51%) / **Protein** 135 g (23%) / **Fat** 68 g (26%) / **Fluid** 128

2400 CALORIE MEAL PLAN

DAY 6

Breakfast
7:00 AM

skim milk with calcium	1 Cup(s)	86 cal
drinking water	2 Cup(s)	0 cal
bananas	1 small	90 cal
whole wheat bread	2 slice	200 cal
almond butter	2 Tbsp	200 cal

MEAL TOTAL: Calories 576 cal / Carbs 81 g (54%) / Protein 25 g (17%) / Fat 20 g (29%) / Fluid 26

Snack
10:00 AM

vanilla yogurt, low-fat	6 oz	145 cal
drinking water	2 Cup(s)	0 cal
nectarines	1 fruit	60 cal
triscuit crackers, light salt	6 crackers	120 cal

MEAL TOTAL: Calories 324 cal / Carbs 58 g (68%) / Protein 13 g (15%) / Fat 7 g (17%) / Fluid 25

Lunch
12:00 PM

chopped kale salad with chicken	1 serving	262 cal
whole wheat dinner rolls	2 roll	149 cal
iced tea, green	16 fl oz	0 cal
butter, no salt	1/2 Tbsp	51 cal

MEAL TOTAL: Calories 462 cal / Carbs 38 g (32%) / Protein 38 g (32%) / Fat 19 g (36%) / Fluid 22

Snack
3:00 PM

drinking water	2 Cup(s)	0 cal
apples	1 small	55 cal
nut and raisin granola bars	1 bar	127 cal
pretzel sticks, no salt	40 pretzels	117 cal

MEAL TOTAL: Calories 299 cal / Carbs 57 g (74%) / Protein 6 g (7%) / Fat 7 g (19%) / Fluid 19

Dinner
6:00 PM

salmon, cooked	3 oz	130 cal
drinking water	2 Cup(s)	0 cal
wild rice, cooked	1 1/2 Cup(s)	248 cal
butter, no salt	1/2 Tbsp	51 cal
summer squash, no salt, boiled	3/4 cup	27 cal
mixed vegetables, frozen no salt, boiled	1 Cup(s)	59 cal

MEAL TOTAL: Calories 516 cal / Carbs 70 g (54%) / Protein 35 g (26%) / Fat 12 g (20%) / Fluid 31

DAY 6 TOTAL: Calories 2,178 cal / **Carbs** 305 g (54%) / **Protein** 116 g (21%) / **Fat** 64 g (25%) / **Fluid** 123

2400 CALORIE MEAL PLAN

DAY 7

Breakfast
7:00 AM

whole wheat bread	2 slice	200 cal
whole eggs, poached	2 large	143 cal
orange juice	1 Cup(s)	112 cal
drinking water	1 Cup(s)	0 cal
butter, no salt	1/2 Tbsp	51 cal
blackberries	1 Cup(s)	62 cal

MEAL TOTAL: Calories 568 cal / **Carbs** 80 g (54%) / **Protein** 26 g (17%) / **Fat** 19 g (29%) / **Fluid** 22

Snack
10:00 AM

hummus, lower sodium	2 Tbsp	52 cal
baby carrots	20 large	105 cal
drinking water	2 Cup(s)	0 cal
pretzel sticks, no salt	40 pretzels	117 cal

MEAL TOTAL: Calories 274 cal / **Carbs** 54 g (76%) / **Protein** 7 g (11%) / **Fat** 4 g (13%) / **Fluid** 26

Lunch
12:00 PM

turkey breast, roasted	4 oz	154 cal
drinking water	2 Cup(s)	0 cal
tomatoes	1/2 Cup(s)	16 cal
dijon mustard	2 tsp	10 cal
romaine lettuce	4 leaf	4 cal
olive oil, mayonnaise, light	2 tsp	33 cal
whole wheat tortillas	2 tortilla	254 cal

MEAL TOTAL: Calories 472 cal / **Carbs** 43 g (36%) / **Protein** 43 g (37%) / **Fat** 14 g (27%) / **Fluid** 23

Snack
3:00 PM

vanilla yogurt, low-fat	8 oz	193 cal
drinking water	2 Cup(s)	0 cal
strawberries	1 cup	53 cal
granola oat cereal, low-fat	1/2 Cup(s)	63 cal

MEAL TOTAL: Calories 309 cal / **Carbs** 58 g (71%) / **Protein** 13 g (17%) / **Fat** 4 g (12%) / **Fluid** 27

Dinner
6:00 PM

brussels sprouts, no salt, boiled	1 Cup(s)	28 cal
drinking water	2 Cup(s)	0 cal
quinoa, cooked	1 Cup(s)	222 cal
chicken, boneless, roasted	4 oz	189 cal
butter, no salt	1/2 Tbsp	51 cal

MEAL TOTAL: Calories 491 cal / **Carbs** 45 g (36%) / **Protein** 39 g (32%) / **Fat** 17 g (32%) / **Fluid** 25

DAY 7 TOTAL: Calories 2,113 cal / **Carbs** 279 g (52%) / **Protein** 128 g (24%) / **Fat** 59 g (24%) / **Fluid** 124

FOOD EXCHANGE LIST

FORGE // FOOD EXCHANGE LIST

FRUIT 50 CALORIES	VEGGIES 50 CALORIES	PROTEIN 50 CALORIES	CARBS 50 CALORIES
APPLE 100g Protein // .2g Carbs // 13g Fat // 0.1g	**ANY SALAD GREENS** 200g Protein // 6g Carbs // 8g Fat // 0.8g	**96% LEAN GROUND BEEF-COOKED** 30g Protein // 9g Carbs // 0g Fat // 1g	**BROWN RICE-COOKED** 45g Protein // 1g Carbs // 10g Fat // 0.4
BANANA 60g Protein // 0.6g Carbs // 13g Fat // 0.1g	**ASPARAGUS** 250g Proteins // 5g Carbs // 10g Fat // 0.3g	**93% LEAN GROUND BEEF-COOKED** 25g Protein // 7g Carbs // 0g Fat // 2.5g	**BUTTERNUT SQUASH-UNCOOKED** 110g Protein // 1g Carbs // 13g Fat // 0.1g
BLACKBERRIES 120g Protein // 1.6g Carbs // 12g Fat // 0.1	**BROCCOLI** 140g Protein // 5g Carbs // 12g Fat // 1g	**99% LEAN GROUND TURKEY-COOKED** 40g Protein // 12g Carbs // 0g Fat // 0.4g	**GLUTEN FREE-PASTA-DRY** 15g Protein // 1g Carbs // 12g Fat // 0.2g
BLUEBERRIES 90g Protein // 0.6g Carbs // 13g Fat // 0.2g	**BRUSSEL SPROUTS** 100g Protein // 3.4g Carbs // 9g Fat // 0.3g	**93% LEAN GROUND TURKEY-COOKED** 25g Protein // 7g Carbs // 0g Fat // 2.5g	**GOLD POTATO-COOKED** 30g Protein // 1g Carbs // 13g Fat // 0g
GRAPES 75g Protein // 0.5g Carbs // 13g Fat // 1g	**CAULIFLOWER** 200g Protein // 4g Carbs // 10g Fat // 0.6g	**95% LEAN GROUND CHICKEN-COOKED** 30g Protein // 7g Carbs // 0g Fat // 3g	**KODIAK POWERCAKES-DRY** 15G Protein // 4 g Carbs // 9g Fat // 0.5g

FRUIT 50 CALORIES	VEGGIES 50 CALORIES	PROTEIN 50 CALORIES	CARBS 50 CALORIES
GRAPEFRUIT 165g Protein // 1g Carbs // 13g Fat // 0.1g	**CELERY** 250G Protein // 2g Carbs // 10g Fat // 0.7g	**CHICKEN BREAST-BONELESS SKINLESS-COOKED** 40g Protein // 12g Carbs // 0g Fat // 0.5	**OATMEAL-DRY** 15G Protein // 2g Carbs // 10g Fat // 1g
NECTARINE 120G Protein // 1.3g Carbs // 13g Fat // 0.3g	**GREEN BEANS** 150G Protein // 1g Carbs // 4g Fat // 0.2g	**COTTAGE CHEESE 1%** 65G Protein // 9g Carbs // 2g Fat // 0.5g	**QUAKER CARAMEL RICE CAKE - 1 RICE CAKE** Protein // 1g Carbs // 11g Fat // 0g
ORANGE 110G Protein // 1g Carbs // 13g Fat // 0.1g	**MUSHROOMS** 200G Protein // 6g Carbs // 7g Fat // 0.6g	**COTTAGE CHEESE 2%** 60G Protein // 7g Carbs // 2.5 Fat // 1	**QUINOA-COOKED** 40G Protein // 2g Carbs // 9g Fat // 1g
PEACH 135G Protein // 1g Carbs // 13g Fat // 0.3g	**ONIONS** 100G Protein // 1.1g Carbs // 9g Fat // 0.9g	**EGG WHITES-100% LIQUID** 95G Protein // 10g Carbs // 0g Fat // 1.5g	**SWEET POTATO-COOKED** 15G Protein // 1g Carbs // 11g Fat // 0g
PEAR 90G Protein // 0.3g Carbs // 14g Fat // 1g	**PEPPERS-GREEN, RED, YELLOW** 250G Protein // 4g Carbs // 10g Fat // 0.4	**GREEK YOGURT-NONFAT PLAIN** 90G Protein // 10g Carbs // 3.5g Fat // 0g	**TORTILLA-CORN (MISSION)** 1 TORTILLA Protein // 1g Carbs // 10g Fat // 1g

FRUIT 50 CALORIES	VEGGIES 50 CALORIES	PROTEIN 50 CALORIES	CARBS 50 CALORIES
PLUM 115G Protein // 0.3g Carbs // 14g Fat // 1g	**SNOW PEA PODS** 100G Protein // 3g Carbs // 8g Fat // 0.2g	**PORK CHOPS-** **BONELESS SKINLESS-** **COOKED** 30G Protein // 8g Carbs // 0g Fat // 2g	**WHITE RICE-COOKED** 45G Protein // 1g Carbs // 12g Fat // 0g
POMEGRANATE 60G Protein // 1g Carbs // 12g Fat // 0.7g	**SPAGHETTI SQUASH** 150G Protein // 0.9g Carbs // 11g Fat // 0.9g	**SHRIMP-COOKED** 60G Protein // 12g Carbs // 0.1g Fat // 0g	**WHITE POTATO-COOKED** 15G Protein // 1g Carbs // 12g Fat // 0.1g
RASPBERRIES 100G Protein // 1.2g Carbs // 12g Fat // 0.6g	**SPINACH** 200G Protein // 6g Carbs // 8g Fat // 0.8g	**TURKEY BACON-** 1 ½ SLICES Protein // 9g Carbs // 0g Fat // 2g	**WHOLE WHEAT PASTA-DRY** 15G Protein // 2g Carbs // 10g Fat // 0.3g
STRAWBERRIES 165G Protein // 1g Carbs // 13g Fat // 0.5g	**SUMMER SQUASH** 300G Protein // 4g Carbs // 10g Fat // 0.6g	**TUNA-CANNED IN WATER** 65G Protein // 12g Carbs // 0g Fat // 0.3g	**UNCLE BENS CREAM** **OF RICE-DRY** 15G Protein // 0.7g Carbs // 12g Fat // 0g
WATERMELON 175G Protein // 1g Carbs // 13g Fat // 0.2g	**ZUCCHINI** 300G Protein // 4g Carbs // 10g Fat // 0.6g	**TURKEY DELI MEAT-NO HONEY** 60G Protein // 12g Carbs // 0g Fat // 1g	**UNCLE BENS CREAM** **OF WHEAT-DRY** 15G Protein // 2g Carbs // 10g Fat // 0g

ACKNOWLEDGEMENTS

It is my sincere hope the contents of this book have helped you organize a meaningful approach to habit alteration. We all have our unique life situations, fears, and limitations.

We also have the power to work towards our potential by overcoming these fears and challenging our limiting beliefs. I wish you success in your journey to improve and create a sustainable fitness and nutrition lifestyle.

I would like to acknowledge a few folks who have given support, challenged me, or contributed to my life and career in a meaningful way.

To my mother, Laura Parker.
To my late grandmother, Francis George.
To Heather Turning.
To all my siblings: Mark Parker, Matthew Parker, Michaela Velarde-Parker, my adopted Brazilian brother, Renato Guerra. Plus, their significant others, Daisy Parker, Rebecca Parker, Alfredo Velarde, and Aline Guerra, my adopted Brazilian sister.

To the Forge coaching team and contractors who have contributed greatly to the Forge brand: Carrie Gilbert, Milly Nuñez, Tate Odell, Samantha Ostarello, Cameron Lemieux, Serena Starks, Stacie Ringleb, Lori Frech, Jennifer McCalib, Anna Bartholemy, Heather Turning with Turning Heads Designs, Justin Doyle, and Chris Smearing. And finally, our advertising and brand development team at Van Bram,

To those who supported my professional carrer prior to Forge: Bobby Harasin, Sal Di Stafano, Jeff Skelton, Dean Pappous, Mark Polli, Regi Allison, Ben Rathe, James Garing, Onome Ojo, Don Lynd, Gary and Deborah Seeger – I thank you all.

Made in the USA
Columbia, SC
05 May 2023

16136466R00211